CAREGIVER 2.0

From Burnout to Powerhouse

Meriam Boldewijn

Dedication to my husband Martin and my brother Patrick.

These two gentlemen have a lot of strength. They've been through many medical challenges but never gave up. They needed help, and I did the best I could with the knowledge I had. When I felt tired, exhausted, and helpless, I needed to be reminded that they didn't ask to be in this situation. I needed support too, and thankfully, I got that from family and friends. Being supported felt like a warm blanket on my skin. Caregiving is hard, and you simply can't do it alone.

I learned many lessons while being the caregiver for Martin and Patrick. Not only did I learn how to take care of them, but I also learned more about myself and grew personally. During those tough times, the question "Why Me" came to my mind very often. As I'm writing this, a big smile comes to my face because now I can say: "Why Not Me."

Thank you, Martin and Patrick. The compassion I learned from being your caregiver inspired me to become a coach for other caregivers across the globe.

TABLE OF CONTENTS

I Am 1

Foreword... 3

Letter to Caregivers... 6

Introduction... 8

Possibility 27

Asking For Help... 44

Scheduling And Organizing... 85

Self-Care 98

Social Connection 124

Review And Reimagine 139

Conclusion: 143

Letter to Martin 145

Letter from Patrick 147

P.S. 148

About the Author 149

Connect with us 150

Resources 151

I AM

I am from a mother who used a calabash and fresh herbs when her child had a fever;

I am from chewing gum, so my mom could fill the holes in the roof with it to prevent me from getting wet when it rained;

I am from parents who told me: Meriam, You Are Enough!

I am from a place where the synagogue and the mosque are neighbors who share traditional food on national holidays;

I am from a place where Christmas, Ied ul fitre, Diwali are national holidays;

I am from eating roti, bami, fried yuca with fish, rice with black beans;

I am from young boys standing on the corner of the street watching those beautiful young ladies passing by and finally saying… ppsssttt, that is immediately followed by rolling eyes and sounds of kissing teeth;

I am from swinging the hips from left to right on kaseko music; I am also from a place of wooden shoes, windmills, canals, bicycles, the creamy Edam and salty Gouda cheese, beautiful tulips, Van Gogh and Rembrandt, and wearing an orange outfit on King's Day.

1

FOREWORD

I had the honor of taking care of my late wife who died of breast cancer. And now as Meriam's husband, it is strange to realize that I am the person receiving care.

My doctor didn't tell me back in 1999 that my kidneys were deteriorating until it was so bad that dialysis was the only option. I started with peritoneal dialysis in 2001, but after many episodes of peritonitis, I had to switch to hemodialysis. When I started with hemodialysis in 2002, I could travel by myself to and from the hospital, but after a couple of months, my physical health deteriorated very fast. Meriam started driving me to and picking me up after dialysis.

One of the doctors told me that I could be a candidate for a kidney-pancreas transplant. This could increase the quality of my life. I loved the idea; it sounded like music to my ears, and the doctor arranged an interview with a specialist in another hospital.

From that specialist, I learned that diabetics with kidney failure on dialysis have a limited life expectancy. He asked me if I could do some tests to see if I was eligible for transplant surgery. After the tests, I could still say no to the surgery even if I was eligible. I agreed, and I passed all the severe physical and medical tests.

During those days, Meriam was doing more and more in our lives because my time was consumed by my job, dialysis, and recovering from dialysis. Since my condition was going downhill, her caregiving was going uphill.

One day, after one of the treatments, we went to a birthday party at a friend's house. I'll never forget the frightened faces of all the people when I came in and fell face forward on a bed in a guestroom. The next day I realized that my days were numbered, and I probably had about twelve to eighteen months left if I didn't do the kidney-pancreas transplant surgery. Meriam and I talked about it, and I called the specialist to say that we wanted to go for the surgery. I say "we" because I couldn't have done this alone.

More than one year later, when I opened my eyes for the first time on November 24th, 2003, I saw the two smiling faces: Meriam and my mom, and I realized that our future would last more than twelve to eighteen months.

Never give up hope!

Love you Meriam.

-Martin

TO: ALL CAREGIVERS

Address: Anywhere in the world

Date: Today

Re: Thank you!

Dear Caregiver,

You are taking care of your loved one: your spouse, partner, sibling, parent, or friend. You're humble and I know that you need to have a lot of courage, strength, and patience. I appreciate you for what you're doing because you are not obligated to do it. The reason why you're doing it is because of the love towards your loved one.

Caregiving is challenging; both mentally and physically. Most of the time your mind and body are not in balance. While your friends and family are enjoying life, you chose to stay home with your loved one. Sometimes you don't feel appreciated, because very often you don't get help. You are up till late at night and the next day you start with a "low battery" because you didn't have enough sleep.

I want you to know that you are loved by me. Despite the hard work, I ask you to take good care of yourself, both mentally and physically, because you are needed more than you realize. Reaching out, asking questions, asking for help, and maintaining self-care is not a selfish act but important for your well-being as well as the person you care for. Yes, read that again!

If you have difficulties in the areas of asking for help, communication, and maintaining self-care, I'm more than willing to teach you how to do it. Promise yourself that if you're stuck, you'll read this letter and rise again.

Caregiver, I thank you for what you're doing. And please know that you are worthy of a wonderful life too!

Warm regards,

Fellow caregiver
Meriam Boldewijn

INTRODUCTION

> *Dear Caregiver,*
>
> *Who do you belong to?*

I belong to the Universe. Why? Because I Ask, Believe, and Receive. This is how the Universe works, and I am so grateful that every day I trust and understand it better. I'm not there yet. You might not be there either. Begin where you are. I also belong to my husband, family members, and friends. I don't know everything, but what I do know is that I can and will help others with the knowledge that I have. I Ask, I Believe, I Receive.

As you're reading this book, I invite you to choose a space in or outside your home where there is more energy, more peace; a positive environment.

In September of 2020, all we could hear on the news was Covid-19. September 22 was our 15th wedding anniversary, and we decided at the last minute to celebrate in the Douro Valley in Portugal. Martin and I were addicted to traveling, and we were excited, but not afraid. We wore our face masks while traveling, and the two-hour flight to Porto went very well.

It was an hour's drive from Porto Airport to our hotel in the Douro Valley. The hotel was on top of a mountain and surrounded by vineyards, lemon trees, and orange trees. There was a nice pool outside, and I could tell by the noise that the birds were making, that they were having the time of their life. The hotel was on the Douro river, and across the river, there was a road and a railway. Once in a while, you could hear the traffic or the train. Other than that, it was quiet. Our room had a balcony, and I used to sit there in the evening watching the uncountable stars and enjoying the quietness.

We spent nine days at this beautiful hotel, and we took a nice rest, celebrated our anniversary, and I worked on this book. Me-time for myself and my husband was our priority. Together we were grateful that we could enjoy the rest, the surroundings, and great traditional food from the Viseu area in Portugal. Today Martin is physically healthy, but it wasn't always like this.

In the summer of 1999, Martin and I had just moved to our new home, and we were so happy. We were enjoying the quietness of the neighborhood.

Martin is a 6.4 ft white, bald, and slender man with green eyes, a firm nose, not too thin lips, and what I love is his dimple on his left cheek and the one on his chin. Yes, Martin is a handsome guy. He had a recurring doctor's appointment once every four months to check if there needed to be medical adjustments for his diabetes. We sat down, and the doctor looked at Martin's file.

"Martin, the values of your kidneys have dropped very much. They only function at 17%. You have to stay in the hospital for more examinations."

Martin squeezed my hand, and that's when I knew he was mad.

"You should have told me earlier. Why do I hear this now; why haven't you told me earlier that I have kidney failure!

I was stunned and did not move! What does kidney failure mean? 17% is very low, so what's the next step? While I was thinking about these questions, Martin was still talking to the doctor. Yes, it was not fair to NOT tell your patient that his kidneys were deteriorating. Yes, he should have told Martin earlier to prepare him for what was coming. I was angry, steam was coming out of my ears. What was going to happen to Martin?

When we left the room, I told Martin that I would go home to get some clothes for him, call his mother, and come back. I remember that I had to take the subway, and suddenly, while waiting for the metro, I started crying.

I called my sister, who lived twenty minutes away from us, and told her what had happened. She didn't hesitate and told me that she would spend the night with me at home. I felt a sense of relief because this was the first time I would experience Martin being in the hospital.

I felt unsettled and alone; my hubby wasn't home. We had two old cats, a male Abyssinian and a calico. They always came to the front door when they heard our keys in the slot. I won't forget their eyes when they saw me alone. *Where's the boss? Where's the one I can sleep on the chest? I want to cuddle.* They kept meowing; they felt something was wrong. I cuddled with them and told them that their boss would be home soon.

Martin's mom was in shock when I notified her that her son was suffering from kidney failure.

I went back to the hospital by car, and when I entered the room, I saw Martin sitting on the hospital bed. My heart broke; I felt helpless and enraged because the doctor didn't notify him earlier. It just wasn't fair!

At the same time, I thought:

"Meriam, let it go. Focus on Martin and ask as many questions as you can think of to the doctor."

A few days went by, and Martin had some medical examinations. When they were done, the doctor decided that, since there was no nephrologist in that hospital, Martin's file would be transferred to a hospital where they have more knowledge of kidney failure. And that's when the long journey of kidney failure, dialysis, and transplant started.

Fast forward to today, Martin is doing physically well. We have been through a lot, but the connection between us is stronger than ever before. We are soulmates, and we stay in our power and live in harmony.

We are careful around the issues of Covid-19, but we try to live our lives as much as we can and don't live in fear. I had a cold in December 2020 and went to test for Covid-19. The outcome was negative. I was not in fear because I keep hope alive. I can do that because hope was an early lesson in Surinam.

I remember our house as being a safe place. It had three bedrooms, one bath, one toilet, a small living room, and a small kitchen. The floor was made of cement. No carpeting. There was no air conditioning. The only way air could enter or leave the rooms was through the shutters. The roof was a tin roof. I loved the sound of the raindrops on the roof, especially at night. It made me relax and fall asleep quickly. Mom loved flowers in the garden; especially the roses and "faja lobi," which means ardent love. It's the favorite flower of most Surinamese people and comes in red, white, yellow, and orange. The small fruits that look like tiny grapes, taste sweet and are a true treat for the hummingbirds. In the front of the house, we had a beautiful "krere-krere" (*Caesalpinia Pulcherrima*) plant. The dragonflies love this plant, and I ate the fruits that look and taste like legumes.

We lived in our cozy house from the moment I was born, and I remember sharing a room with one of my sisters and brother. Mom, dad, and five children in a three-bedroom house. It was busy sometimes, but my parents made sure that it was manageable. We were happy, had food and clean clothes every day, and those were the most important things. I also have a sister and brother from another mama, and they called my mother "auntie" and "mom". I've always had a special bond with each of my siblings. It was very comforting for me to know that; besides my parents, I could ask questions of any of them. Now that I think back, I'm reminded that asking for help was not a problem for me as a child. As a caregiver, when I sometimes think if I should ask for help, I think of the time when I just did it. The strength and support of my family helped me grow up.

Dear Caregiver,
As a child, did you find it easy to ask for help? Did you watch other people ask for help too?

When I was eight years old, I imagined God could provide my family with money to buy a new roof for our house. You see, the roof was leaking, and every time it would rain, mom called my siblings and me to chew gum. I can hear you thinking: WHY chewing gum? This gum she used to fill the holes in the tin roof so we wouldn't get wet when it rained. What a clever woman!

Mom never stopped believing in God, and neither did I. He gave mom the knowledge to manage money, even though she only finished primary school. God gave dad the strength to work at the harbor until his retirement, even though he had a heart condition.

He played a card game with friends for money. In 1981, he rented a small place where he organized card games for a small group. He gave all the money he earned to mom, and he could go on his knees, but she would never give him the money back. Within two years, mom and dad saved enough money to build a new house with four bedrooms, two bathrooms, and a solid roof. Consistency, belief, and hard work paid off!

I told you before that my mom was a strong and clever woman. Her mom died when she was only seven and she grew up with her four siblings. My grandpa had to take care of his five children, losing his wife at just thirty-five. It was a tough time. Each day grandpa had to bring children from the district to school. Via the river, on the boat, that was grandpa's job. He was in church every Sunday and knew the nuns, priests, and other people from church. One day a nun told grandpa there was a Chinese family in the capital with two boys and one deaf-mute girl who was looking for a girl of the same age as their daughter to join the family. Mom was a good fit and had finished primary school. Her youngest sister was seven years old; the older sister was fifteen and was the one who did the mommy tasks (cooking and cleaning) when grandma died, and the boys helped grandpa with heavy work in and around the house and in the field.

I don't know exactly how it all went, but mom ended up with that Chinese family at the age of twelve.

Mom had a roof above her head, clean clothes, and food every day. But she didn't go to school. Mom helped the Chinese couple with the household and their deaf-mute daughter. She missed grandpa and her siblings very much. It makes me cry when I think of how I would feel if I had to leave my family home at that age. Mom was not able to call them and had to wait until school holidays to play and laugh with them. Although miles apart their love and connection remained strong.

I remember my mom telling me the story of how she met my dad. She was sitting on her balcony when a handsome guy went by on his bike. He waved at her and that's how it all started. They fell in love, and on July 21, 1954, they got married. At the age of twenty-one, she left the Chinese family and a whole new chapter started.

This clever woman probably learned how to save money in the first twelve years of her life when she saw how grandpa worked hard to take care of his children after his wife died. Or she learned how to save money when she was with the Chinese family and promised herself that she would make sure that her kids could go to high school and beyond.

Mom had a very close relationship with her siblings, despite the circumstances, and that's something I will never forget. It not only inspired but also nourished the relationship I have with my siblings today.

I've always had a close relationship with my mom. She was such a beautiful black woman, 5'4 ft of height with a US size 20/22, big breasts, and firm upper arms. When she laughed, you couldn't help laughing; it was contagious.

As a seven-year-old child, on a hot day, I had a fever. Mom was worried, but she knew what to do and went into the garden to pick some leaves; the "fever leaves"; in Surinamese it's called "korsoe wiri".

Mom mashed those leaves in a big calabash, added water, and let it sit for at least half an hour. The calabash mom used is a bottle gourd with hard hollow fruit of the calabash tree (*Crescentia cujete*). The fruit is also used to make utensils, containers, and musical instruments. Mom told me to wear my "pangi," which is a piece of African print fabric that you tie around your body. When the water and fever leaves were ready, she called me:

"Meriam, please come over here."

She was already standing in the sandy backyard
with the calabash and fever leaves in her hand.

Dear Caregiver,
Even if you don't know what a calabash is, do you remember
something tender from your childhood? Like when a ma or
grandma tended to your physical being?

I could hear the birds whistling, as the leaves of
the trees went from left to right in the wind, while the sun
was shining very bright. I was not feeling ok and didn't
like the idea of getting cold water on my head. But I knew
mom was worried and wanted to help. When I stood in
front of her, she told me that we would pray first. Ask
Mother Earth for guidance and relief from the fever. We
started praying. Remember, I did not feel well, but when
we were praying, I felt the strength of mom's voice. The
way she was praying convinced me that I would be ok,
and that strengthened me although I was shivering, and
could barely stand on my feet. When we were done
praying, mom looked at me and said: "you're going to be
fine, BELIEVE it!". And I did.

When she poured the first few drops on my head,
it felt like ice on my skin. I started shivering more while
mom kept pouring. I can still remember the fresh and
intense smell of those leaves. She made sure that the
leaves touched my skin, so their elements could enter my
body through my pores. The two-minute ritual seemed

like forever to me. When we were done, mom took me to the bathroom and took off the wet pangi.

Dear Caregiver,
Do you ever anticipate the moment of caregiving? Do you know the feeling of relief?

She handed me a towel to dry my skin and I put on some clothes. Within one hour the fever was gone!

The way she took care of me made me feel safe and loved. She not only taught me that nature has its strength; she also taught me that taking care of someone you love is necessary, both mentally and physically. Her knowledge and beliefs were so strong, and I picked up her energy.

Mom took care of me, but Mother Earth took care of both of us.

After my 10th birthday, I suffered from belly pain. It became such a severe pain that my mom took me to the doctor, and he redirected us to the hospital, where they found out that I had an umbilical hernia. I needed surgery, and the doctor didn't want to wait too long. I was scared because I never had any surgery, and the idea that they would cut in my body made me feel nauseous. On January 19, 1981, I had surgery. I can vaguely remember my mother's youngest sister standing at my bedside, but I was too sleepy to talk. Her smile comforted me and assured me that although my belly hurt, I was going to be ok. The next day when mom and dad visited me in the hospital, I could tell by their happy faces that they had great news. They told me that the doctor said that I was going to be fine, and also that I became an auntie earlier that day. A couple of months ago, my sister had announced that she was pregnant. I was excited and hoped that it would be a girl. I imagined combing her hair, doing her nails, and all the fun things we could do. I was so happy and couldn't wait to go back home.

When it was safe to travel with the baby, and my sister came to our place, I was so excited to see and hold my beautiful baby niece for the first time. I had a huge band-aid and needed to sit in a certain position, so her weight wouldn't hurt my belly. I was a very proud ten-year-old auntie. I helped by washing and feeding the baby whenever there was a chance. And so, I began my caregiving role, even though I didn't know what that word meant. Often, we are caregiving without even knowing it.

By the time I turned nineteen, I was an auntie to three nephews I helped mom look after when their parents were at work. In taking care of those children, I could offer mom some relief. I remember how much she enjoyed ironing; in a way, it was her me-time. I think it was the swinging from left to right that calmed her. It was a moment where she could breathe.

Mom only allowed me to take care of the kids if I had my homework done and had taken my siesta. She took care of me so I could take care of her. So beautiful...

At that age, I still didn't realize that I was a caregiver or what the word caregiver meant.

Lots of caregivers take care of their children, grandchildren, nieces, and nephews.

Dear Caregiver,
Do you have an early memory of caregiving? Are you committed to your nieces or nephews, and do you feel stuck and cornered sometimes?

My nephews brought so much love, happiness, and laughter. Imagine me having one baby in a wrap on my back and chasing a toddler who escaped to the backyard or discovering two toddlers spilling mom's coconut oil on the ground and sliding continuously because of it. Now that I look back, I just don't know how I did it. But I'm grateful that I could see them grow up until it was time for me to move to the Netherlands.

I've been in the Netherlands for thirty years now.

Surinam was a colony of the Netherlands until November 25, 1975. So, when I was born in 1970, I officially had Dutch nationality. My image of the

Netherlands was: cold weather, wearing layers, grey skies, being inside your house for months. No, thank you! But my mom and dad had a conversation with me at the age of nineteen because the economy in Surinam wasn't what it had been before. My parents suggested that I move to have a better future. When I talked to my best friend (BFF), she mentioned that her parents also suggested moving to the Netherlands.

I gave it a serious thought, but the idea of trading the nice warm weather still made me feel unhappy. A couple of weeks later, mom and dad asked me again and when they saw my hesitance, they suggested that I should at least give it a try. I told them that I would go on holiday, but for only two weeks. It was June 1991, and thirty years later, I am still on holiday in the Netherlands.

I remember wearing jeans, white sneakers, and a pink-white striped polo and jeans jacket on the day I flew to the Netherlands. I left home, my family and baby nephew, who was seven months old. I took care of him when my sister was at work. My parents who were visiting my brother and sisters in the Netherlands would pick me up at the airport. The idea of joining them was equally scary and exciting. I knew they would look after me but leaving home felt heavy on my heart.

I left my home on June 10, 1991; everything I knew, my comfort zone, my safety net stayed behind. That heartache I felt leaving my baby nephew who was so attached to me, was nearly unbearable. Imagine me sweeping the carport every morning while carrying this baby in a cloth tied on my back. He couldn't talk yet, but my sister told me that when I left, he looked for me in the house. He crawled to my bedroom to see if I was there and came back with questioning eyes: where is auntie?

I met my BFF at the airport. It was a straight flight of approximately nine hours, and I slept a bit, but couldn't help thinking about the safe place I left. I was grateful that my parents were on holiday in the Netherlands because if I had to leave them in Surinam, I don't know if I would go to the airport.

Before landing, the captain told the passengers that the weather was great; 13C/55F. I looked at my BFF and said:

"I think he made a mistake; it's June, almost summer, so it must be 31C/87F, right?"

My BFF laughed because she had been to the Netherlands before. She said, "you might want to close the buttons of your jacket."

"Nah, I'm ok."

We landed, and when we got out of the plane, I didn't feel the cold yet. The gigantic airport seemed very modern to me. There was a pleasant temperature. I looked at all the fancy shops, restaurants, and all the other travelers. It was so crowded. Where were all these people going?

We went to pick up our luggage, and my BFF reminded me to close my jacket.

"Nah, I'm fine sis."

When we got our luggage, we proceeded to the exit. I saw my parents, sister, and brother-in-law and we hugged and kissed. My sister is ten years older than me and has such a great smile. Her ex-husband is a 6'2 ft tall man with a great sense of humor. To be honest, I was happy I wasn't alone in the Netherlands.

My BFF also met her sister and brother-in-law and we all talked for a minute. But then, we had to split. The distance between me and my BFF was not ten to fifteen minutes anymore, but at least one hour! We could call each other, but we were used to seeing each other. Another moment of sadness. We promised to call, and we all went to the parking garage. When I went outside the airport, I felt the cold wind which surprised me because it was a clear blue sky. Mom told me to close my jacket, and I did; now I understood what my BFF meant.

On the way home, I didn't talk; I was looking at how different the Netherlands was from Surinam. There were no power wires connected to the lamp posts, they drove very fast in two or three lanes next to each other, and the people talked fast. I saw trains, trams, cars, bicyclists, pedestrians; it was all so much. When we got home, I was tired. My sister showed me my room, and I loved it. It had light mint-colored walls, a white bed, and a white closet. They did their best to make it comfortable. I took a shower and went to bed. The time difference with Surinam was five hours, and by the time I was home, it was 5 AM in Surinam.

My two weeks holiday had begun. I was grateful for having my parents with me. The next question was: do I want to live in the Netherlands? The next day I went with mom and dad to visit my sister and her two boys in Amsterdam. She moved to the Netherlands a couple of months earlier. I was so happy to see my nephews who were two and five years old.

Later that day we visited my brother, who also lived in Amsterdam. He had beautiful four-year-old twin girls and a two-year-old boy. I had only seen the girls once when they visited us in Surinam. It felt good being with the family, and I could see that my parents felt rich when they were with their children and grandchildren, both in the Netherlands and Surinam.

After a couple of days, I noticed that I liked being in the Netherlands despite the cold weather. But I didn't like the thought of my parents leaving soon. Dad had a serious conversation with me once more and told me that there is always a way to be with them: there are airplanes! I thought about his words and decided to stay. I had to arrange a lot of paperwork, but because I had Dutch nationality when I was born, I was naturalized.

When I moved to the Netherlands, I had so much support from my family. It made it easier for me to stay in a foreign country. When support is offered, and when hope exists, perhaps it is easier to ask for help.

I know that caregiving can be exhausting. We sometimes keep on going because of the thought that we need to and that there's no choice. But is that true? I think we have a choice. Today I can say that I did what I could with the knowledge I had. I chose to offer help, but I also chose Meriam. I commit to loving myself. If I don't do that, how can I commit to others? Yes, I do believe that I was chosen for this job to learn more about myself. It might be hard sometimes, but have you ever thought about your purpose in this world? For me, caregiving is a service and a mission. But I have to be honest that in those hectic moments, it did not feel that way. I sometimes got mad! Not at my loved one, but the disease! Once again: I did what I could with the knowledge I had. I am proud of myself; for permitting myself to acknowledge how brave I am.

I sincerely hope that you know that you are brave. And if no one told you, please know that I am proud of you and of what you are doing as a caregiver.

In the following chapters, I'm going to guide you on how to commit yourself to imagine <u>possibilities</u>.

Asking for help is also a way of committing to yourself. If I ask for help, then I'm more likely to commit time to myself. If I don't ask for help, I am less likely to take time for myself. I resisted asking for help, not just because I didn't want to bother people, but because I didn't want to look at myself!

You will also read why it is important to schedule and organize. Creating time for yourself is a huge benefit. It was easier for me to take care of my loved one, rather than to do self-care! I'm also going to guide why, how, and when to socially connect with people.

When you're finished reading this book, you will have your Personal Assistant SOS with an extra S for the rest of your life! Anywhere along the way, you can reach out and find me at support@meriamboldewijn.com

I have created a safe space for caregivers like you to strengthen their Personal Assistant SOS (PASOSS).

While working on this, please keep FOLLOW in mind.

Forgive yourself

Be **O**pen-minded

Listen to your gut

Learn new things

See and grab **O**pportunities

Know your **W**orth

POSSIBILITY

What do I need to believe that there is a possibility?

I imagine myself being on the other side from where I currently am. That feeling makes me happy and makes me believe that it's possible. And when I believe it's possible, I am more likely to do my best to make it happen.

Who would have thought we would be able to fly? An airplane makes it possible for people to meet in person. An airplane made it possible for me to fly to Surinam and take care of my mom, so my sister and my niece could have some time for self-care; they could breathe. This same airplane gave me the possibility to go to Curacao after my mom died, and my BFF could take care of me.

I was fifteen years old when my sister took me on my first flight to Curacao. I was so excited and not afraid at all. When you have family in several places on earth, and you can travel, an airplane is often the fastest way to get from home to home in one day.

> *Dear Caregiver,*
> *Have you ever thought of what's possible for you at this moment? Like right NOW!*
> *Or are you afraid to believe in possibilities?*
> *Or are you stuck in impossibility If so, how does that make you feel?*

Could you start writing this affirmation:
I am capable of creating possibilities!

When I reflected on what was possible for Martin or my brother Patrick, I ignored myself. I don't want you to do that. And now, even in the moment of Covid, we find ourselves asking the same question: what is possible for me now?

We sometimes limit what is possible because we are afraid. The Fear of what might happen to our loved one is huge and many times Fear won't give Possibility a chance. I can come up with ten impossibilities before I come up with one possibility.

When I open to possibilities, I create a mindset for change.

For example, Martin and I went on a holiday to Surinam when Martin was on peritoneal dialysis. As much as Martin wanted to go on a diving holiday, that was a big

NO, so neither would a climb on the Himalayas. But there were other possibilities:

- Martin was allowed to fly.
- His peritoneal fluids and medical supplies could be transported to Surinam.
- In case of emergency, there were nephrologists in Surinam and there were daily flights on the route.
- We could stay with my mother, and we knew it was neat and clean.

Instead of looking at what was impossible, we looked for what was possible.

When Martin started with dialysis, I realized that traveling would be different. Traveling would only be possible if we could arrange all necessary medical supplies being delivered at the holiday address when he was on peritoneal dialysis or if we traveled to countries where there were dialysis centers where he could go three times a week to do hemodialysis. I must say that our 14-day holiday trip to Torremolinos, Spain was an awesome experience. This trip was organized by the Kidney Foundation, and we were in a group of approximately 15 people, nurses included. All was taken care of, and the only thing we needed to do was pack our bags and know when the flight left. Torremolinos is a beautiful place. I went to the dialysis center with Martin a couple of times, and after treatment, we went for lunch on the beach. The freshly grilled sardines were yummy, and we enjoyed the clear blue sky, ocean view, sea breeze, and sun. Yeah, what if it all goes well on holiday!

Opening up for possibilities means permitting yourself to travel together or alone. It can also mean permitting yourself to find ways to not be limited by the medical issues of your loved one. You will be amazed to see how much is possible. Things you thought were impossible seem to be possible.

Dear Caregiver,
Do you go on holiday with your loved one so you can also revitalize your energy? With Covid-19, maybe you can rent a home in the woods, would you do that?

We think of possibilities in moments of crisis, pandemic, or emergency. Why? Because of the energy. We know we have to do something. What if we made a habit of thinking about possibilities when we are calm, going to bed at night or in the morning? Instead of when we are freaking out and saying: what can I do to solve this problem?

It's so amazing to meditate on the idea of possibility.

My brother Patrick had a severe stroke that left him almost incapacitated. He could no longer do his daily functions. And there was a time when I had to shower him every day in the hospital. I had never seen him in his full glory before. It left us both feeling embarrassed.

We have a tendency to feel a little awkward inside when posed with something so delicate and intimate; we can sometimes shy away. Although we know the importance of it for the greater good.

I can still see him lying in that bed and not being able to walk or talk. The nurses could freshen him up every day but could shower him only once a week. They did what they could for their patients in the short amount of time they had. Since I've always had a good relationship with him, I asked him if he was ok with me showering him. He mumbled something and looked away. I could see that he felt uncomfortable, and I understood. He had to put aside his dignity because his situation called for it.

I have to be honest that the idea of seeing my brother, a grown man, naked and cleaning him made me feel awkward too. But there was no way I was going to let embarrassment stop me!

I told him that he didn't have to be ashamed of his younger sister taking care of him. Not only that, but his hygiene was also a top priority, and I believed that showering him daily could speed his recovery.

When he agreed, we as a family discussed the possibility of showering him daily with the medical professionals, and they agreed that we could do it as long as we considered the hospital rules. I asked the nurses for a shower bed for the disabled and the dos and don'ts when showering a partially paralyzed person who's connected to an IV and catheter.

Then it was time to start with the showering mission. Patrick's ex-wife, my nephew, and I made sure that he was showered every day. His left hand was working, so I gave him his toothbrush with toothpaste to brush his teeth. Why? He could do it himself.

When I gave him his toothbrush, he looked at me because he wasn't sure what to do. I said:

"Well, you're paralyzed on the right side, and you are right-handed, but your left arm still works, so why don't you give it a try."

The next thing he did was so hilarious: he put the toothbrush backward in his mouth and looked at me again like he wanted to say: "ok, now what?". He knew that he had to put it in his mouth, but he didn't know what to do next. Patrick did brush his teeth with his left hand though.

The nurses and doctors were blown away when they saw Patrick's improvement after one week. And three months after his stroke, he started walking and talking again. What I learned from this experience is that I should always look for possibilities, grab opportunities and that asking for help is ok. At first, it seemed impossible to have conversations with my loved ones. I needed to find out what their needs were. It was also important for me to know what resources were available. Why? Because knowing it would reduce stress, and I wouldn't have to guess.

After Patrick's stroke, he couldn't stay in his apartment any longer; he needed a safe place with facilities for someone who is partially disabled. I didn't know where to start, and I had to check possibilities. The result after checking possibilities is that he got the keys to his new safe place seven months after his stroke. He also got a mobility scooter so he could go to the supermarket on his own; he didn't have to depend on me or other family members. I checked what his needs were, the resources, and what was possible.

Checking possibilities is so important for both the caregiver and their loved one. Once you can think of the possibility for your loved one, you can turn the mirror to yourself. Thinking about small possibilities like having a latte in the afternoon seems ok. But thinking about bigger possibilities somehow seems impossible. We sometimes don't permit ourselves to think big!

When I was young, I never thought I would be on a famous magazine or a social media cover of a magazine. Well, I did, and here I am in this famous Dutch Magazine called *De Margriet*. I am proud as a woman of color to be featured in a full-page article from this magazine:

Because of the Corona crisis, I have gained some weight. I don't know exactly how much because I haven't been on a scale for years. Since I no longer weigh myself, I feel better, and my weight is more stable.

When I met my husband Martin, I was a size EU 38/US 8. Not long after we met, he became seriously ill. He was ill for years and finally underwent a kidney-pancreas transplant. In that time, I gained as much as 30 kilos. I tried all kinds of diets that only made my weight go up and down. That made me sad and insecure.

At one point I asked my husband:

"Do you still love me? My body has changed."

"I just love Meriam."

That gave my self-confidence such a boost.

From that moment on I started saying to myself every day in the mirror:

"You are a beautiful woman with your full lips, your tummy, and wide hips."

When Martin was physically well, we had to go to a party. I couldn't find anything nice in my size.

That's why I started an online store in 2013; exclusively for plus-sizes, with mainly timeless dresses.

I had that store until last year. I was ready for something new. Closing the store was a difficult and emotional decision: I didn't want to abandon my clients. I wanted to continue giving them the confidence I had. There is still a little yellow paper in my home office with the text:

"Did I already tell you that you are a beautiful woman?

I didn't see this coming. This article reminded me again that there are more possibilities than we can imagine or allow ourselves to imagine!

Dear Caregiver,
Do you feel overwhelmed when even thinking about bigger possibilities?

Please don't think of possibilities that increase stress.

Our friends, family, or medical professionals might open up our understanding of possibilities when we don't know how or when we are blocked.

Sometimes I felt like I was blocked when it came to checking possibilities. When I thought of possibilities that might change my life in a good way, that negative chatter in my head immediately said: "NO, that's impossible!". It kept me in my comfort zone. I needed to learn how to deal with it, and every morning when I woke up, I told myself that it is possible to accomplish many things! Stepping out of that comfort zone slowly and focusing on the positive things kept hope alive. I count my blessings and look at what is going right and learn from the things that go wrong.

What I want to ask you is to think of something you would like to do. Even if it's finishing that book, you started reading months ago. Is it possible to finish it? Yes, it is! Why? You started it; you made time to start, right? So, it is possible. You can make it happen.

Start with a simple daily affirmation: I am going to finish that book because I can. If you say this three times a day and believe it, I guarantee you that it will be possible. It won't be overnight, but it will happen!

All the things you want to be possible can be written first. English is not my main language, and I tell myself every single day that I will also help English-speaking caregivers. I never thought that I would write a book. And here I am, encouraging fellow caregivers to think about possibilities that will allow them to stay in their power and live a harmonious life while they take care of their loved ones. I turned Impossible to I'm Possible!

Even now when I find it hard to imagine possibilities I still try.

I slow down with meditation or journaling. Sometimes I want to do tasks in a hurry or all at once, but it doesn't work; I end up with frustration because things usually go wrong.

Another example is that, as much as we would love to, Martin couldn't do a scuba diving holiday when he was on peritoneal dialysis. It was not medically wise. There were a lot of other possibilities, but I couldn't imagine them. And I also didn't permit myself to see them and I held on to the impossibility. I wish I had not made it so hard for myself. We discovered that snorkeling was possible and also fun to do.

There were so many times I didn't imagine possibilities but should have. I was driving every day for months to the hospital when Martin was recovering from the kidney-pancreas transplant surgery. There was another possibility: I could have chosen to go every other day or four days a week because he had other visitors too. If I had done that, it would have given me more time to rest and/or more me-time. I would be calmer; have time to breathe and more ease.

Checking possibilities is a practice and a commitment because, just like asking for help, it will feel weird the first time. And the second time and maybe the third time. Just start doing it, and you will be stunned when you notice how much is possible. Check possibilities for all the things you want to do next week.

Dear Caregiver,
What possibilities exist for you? What small change can you make for more time for yourself today?

Tomorrow is not guaranteed!

One thing I learned is that life can be over in a blink of an eye. What if we told each other more often how much we appreciate one another and spread the love?

It was April 1996, fifteen months after dad's death. I was on holiday in Surinam, and I had planned a party. My sister wasn't feeling well for weeks. She felt like she couldn't breathe sometimes, and we thought that she had a cold. The day after the party I was at home with mom, an aunt of mine, my niece, and my nephew. I was tired and took a nap in the afternoon. I dreamed that the whole family was on a bus on a bridge except for my sister. She went to the other side of the bridge. When I woke up at 3 PM, I told my mom what I had dreamed. She told me that my brother-in-law had taken my sister to the hospital because she had problems breathing. During visiting hours, I went to my sister with mom, who was terrified and shaking with nerves. She was very concerned about her child. When we went into the room, my sister was gasping for air. It was an awful sight. We didn't stay long because she needed to rest; at least that's what we thought.

It was a long fifteen-minute drive home, with no words. When we got home, mom called my sister's daughter and son who were fifteen and nine at that time. She lit a candle, and the four of us prayed. It was around 7 PM when the phone rang: my sister had just died! I will never forget my niece's face when she heard that her mom died. Yelling, crying, screaming… "Not my mom, why MY mom.. tell me it's a bad dream.. please wake me up". Her little brother just stood there, totally dazed about the news. His mommy was gone. While I'm writing this, I relive the moment, and I get goosebumps and tears dribble on my cheeks again.

Tomorrow is not guaranteed!

The next days of my holiday were filled with planning a funeral, taking care of my mom, niece and nephew, and their father who all were devastated. My sister died from a lung embolism. They found out too late. I had seen my mom broken when dad died, but I'd never seen her like this. The look in her eyes said enough, and it broke my heart in a thousand pieces.

> *Dear Caregiver,*
> *If you knew you had 24 hours to live, what would be possible for you? What would you do, and with whom would you spend those 24 hours?*

After the funeral, I had to come back to the Netherlands. During the flight, all I could think of was my mom and family. What to do next. It's not natural to bury your child; it should be the other way around. Time went by, and my niece and nephew spent more time with my mom because their dad often worked for days in the bush of Surinam. They missed their mom very much, and my fifteen-year-old niece took good care of her little brother. The bond between them became more strengthened.

When he graduated from high school, he came over to the Netherlands to study Aviation Technology and stayed with us for five years. We already had my cousin from Surinam with us here at the house; she was studying Psychology. Having those two adults in our home was a blast. We had many great moments, and I know my late sister is happy that we took care of her son.

Dear Caregiver,
I would like you to think of what's possible for you in the next 24 hours. But I also want to encourage you to think about bigger things that you can't even imagine.

When I was at the doctor with Martin and hearing about his 17% kidney functionality, I couldn't have imagined a trip to Torremolinos or Surinam. While being on peritoneal and hemodialysis, Martin and I went on several short holidays. Our thinking about possibilities should not be limited by fear. You are capable of more than you think. Please, don't underestimate that. Allow yourself to think bigger! If you can imagine a bubble bath for yourself, you can also imagine a weekend getaway for yourself.

What I'm asking you is to make thinking of possibilities a habit, and there are two reasons:

1. One month from now you will be able to think about more extensive possibilities.

2. We can inspire possibilities in each other. Ask friends, family, professionals about what's possible for you.

I used to ask myself the question "Why me?" because caregiving was hard. I was running the whole day, spent 95% of my time on caregiving and I had to do it alone. At least, that's what I thought. And now I ask myself, "Why not me?".

Martin and I couldn't go on a diving holiday when he was on peritoneal dialysis; but what was the equivalent or the next best thing? When I found the next best thing, it was better than the impossible. To make it all possible I had to ask for help. I know that some of you are struggling with asking for help, and that's why I dive into this "issue" in the next chapter.

When you open yourself up to the possibility that you can do so much more for YOU than you ever thought, you could allow yourself to dream BIG.

Congratulations! You have started to strengthen the P of your Personal Assistant SOS with an extra S (PASOSS).

Keep FOLLOW in mind.

Forgive yourself

Be **O**pen-minded

Listen to your gut

Learn new things

See and grab **O**pportunities

Know your **W**orth

ASKING FOR HELP

There is always light at the end of the tunnel.

> *Dear Caregiver,*
> *Do you have the courage to see it?*

Asking for help can be incredibly difficult. I know that for many of you, it's not going to be easy to ask for help. Maybe you've asked your family or friends before, and they may not have supported you. If you've asked for help in the past and the answer has been "no", it's much harder to ask again. And there might be moments when you've asked for help as a woman, and it came with expectations. You knew or thought that it would cost you something. You might be afraid to ask for help, but I'm still going to ask you to move through the fear and ask anyway.

When I was eighteen years old, one of my sisters gave birth to a beautiful nine-pound baby boy. A couple of days after giving birth, my sister told mom that she was in pain because of her hemorrhoids. My late sister who was a nurse took a look and told my sister that she had to see the doctor immediately. It was hard breastfeeding her baby because she couldn't sit properly; it was too painful. I felt sorry for both my sister and the baby.

"How can I help her?"

Mom asked me to take my sister to the hospital for her doctor's appointment. She would stay home to take care of the baby and his three-year-old brother until their father came home from work. It was awful to see my sister in that situation and even though she was in such pain, she still breastfed her son. When we talk about it now, she smiles and says: "I had pain in the breast, and pain in the butt, but the love for my son was unconditional."

It was a twenty-minute drive to the hospital, and I think it was the longest drive ever for her. I tried to be careful and avoided holes in the roads as much as I could. When we arrived at the hospital it took her quite some time to walk to the waiting room. I never left her side. The doctor examined the hemorrhoids and said that they were too big a risk for surgery. She suggested she sit in lukewarm water to let them shrink and come back after two or three days.

I was in high school at that time, and I rushed home every day to help with taking care of both the baby and my sister. During the night I helped with feeding the baby the breast milk she had pumped, so she could rest. Mom did as much as she could.

This lasted for weeks until my sister was feeling better to take care of her son properly. In the end, they didn't do surgery because it was not needed anymore. My sister asked me for help, and I was more than willing to do so. I had been a caregiver without even naming it and I loved it.

Dear Caregiver,
At what age did you become a caregiver?

I learned how to drive at the age of sixteen. Dad was driving a new Opel Senator and whenever mom needed to go somewhere, I asked if I could drive at least one part of the journey in this fancy car.

I remember my oldest sister being at home when she went into labor. The midwife came and when it was time to go to the hospital, I asked dad if he was ready to drive his daughter to the hospital. Dad struggled to see his daughter in pain and asked me to drive. My sister, who was busy dealing with the contractions that came every five minutes, really didn't care who brought her to the hospital.

Mom and I helped my sister get in the back seat between two contractions. The midwife told us that she would wait for us at the hospital, and notify the team that we were coming. My sister was huffing away the contractions in the back seat and when we were five minutes away from the hospital she said:

"MOM, I need to POOP."

I will never forget the look on mom's face; her eyes were as big as saucers:

"Oh no baby girl, please don't make dad's car dirty! We're almost there hon."

Mom was frustrated, my sister was in pain and the baby thought: ok I'm ready for the world. Where's the exit? When we got to the hospital, my sister was brought to the delivery room immediately and of course, mom didn't leave her side. Fifteen minutes later the nurse came and told me that I had become an auntie to a beautiful healthy baby boy. I thanked God for giving me the strength and courage to drive my sister safely to the hospital to give birth to her child. And my dad's car was still clean.

> *Dear Caregiver,*
> *Do you remember a serious but still funny and happy*
> *moment?*

In March 1998, I was working as the administrative assistant for a group of an international tax lawyer's firm and Martin joined that group. He was a very nice guy, and I enjoyed being in his presence. One day in summer 1998, my colleague said:

"Meriam, is there something wrong with your eyes?"

I asked her why.

She said: "don't you see that Martin likes you?".

I said: "no bloody way. Are you kidding me?".

She said: "you need to see an optometrist".

That's when I started paying attention to how Martin was talking to me, behaving in my presence. Yes, it was obvious that he liked me.

Martin and I started dating in July 1998, and on September 24, 1998, we went to the beach in Scheveningen, The Hague. It was partly cloudy, a bit windy and while strolling on the beach, we talked about our experiences in life: the death of our loved ones, the joyful moments as kids and adolescents, our first loves, and how he had taken care of his late wife who died of breast cancer one year after their marriage. When it got chilly, we went for a cup of hot chocolate in one of the beach restaurants. The way Martin looked at me made me feel safe, loved and the feeling I had at that moment is that I could be Meriam; no matter what. I could be the Meriam who sometimes speaks Surinamese; a dialect he now understands very well; the Meriam who sometimes needs to thank Mother Earth with her calabash and water, the Meriam who dances to traditional music, the Meriam who can't help spilling food on her breast in a 3-star restaurant. That's when I knew I wanted to spend the rest of my life with Martin. Mutual respect is the anchor for our relationship.

We both had our apartments, but since Martin lived close to the office, we spent more time together at his place. We traveled to and from work together every day, and before we even realized it, within two months we were living together. People asked me why I moved in so quickly with a guy I had been dating for a short time, but it simply felt good, and I trusted my gut. In the first year that we were together, we traveled a lot; both of us are addicted to traveling.

But what I would like to share with you is that there was a time when traveling was not a priority or a possibility for us. I remember a day back in 2000. Martin suffered from kidney failure due to his diabetes, but he was not on dialysis yet. We had sold both our apartments and bought a beautiful house in a quiet area not far from the busy city. On this day, we had some guests and Martin made some fresh coffee. When he put it on the table, I noticed a strange look in his eyes, and I told our guests: "I have to call the paramedics now! I've never seen this look in his eyes".

I talked to Martin, but he didn't react anymore. He sat straight up and just stared. I told him that I had to measure his blood sugar because I thought it was very low. Martin didn't cooperate and made a fist. I was concerned, nervous and after asking a couple of times he still refused to open his hand. I didn't give up and whispered slowly in his ear:

"Please, open your fist so I can measure your blood sugar."

In the meantime, we were waiting for the paramedics. Since this area was newly built, and I wasn't sure if they would find our home right away, I asked one of the guests to go outside and look out for them. Martin finally opened his hand, so I could measure his blood sugar. It was so low the monitor couldn't give an accurate reading. The first thing that crossed my mind is, OMG he will go into a diabetic coma if the paramedics don't arrive here soon. I started praying and asking for strength to guide us through this difficult moment. Thankfully, after five minutes two male paramedics came in, and I told them that I already measured his blood sugar and that it was so low the monitor couldn't give an accurate reading.

"Thank you so much for doing this. We will insert the IV with the glucose right away."

Applying the IV was not easy because Martin was so strong and wouldn't cooperate. The paramedics held both Martin's hands, two guests were sitting on his legs, and I was whispering in his ear to comfort him. That poor man didn't know what he was doing. The only thing I could think of was, if he goes into a coma now, I will lose him! My heart was beating so fast I thought it would jump out of my body. The adrenaline was racing through my veins, I had sweat on my forehead, but I needed to focus on Martin.

After a few minutes, it felt like hours at that moment, they were able to apply the IV and Martin said:

"What happened?"

"Oh my gosh, he's back!"

I was relieved, but at the same time, I was concerned that this might happen again. I didn't sleep that night, because I was constantly watching him and afraid that he might not wake up.

Dear Caregiver,
What was the scariest moment in your life, and how did you ask for help?

Months went by and the doctor prepared us for dialysis. Martin tried to postpone it as long as possible, but after our trip to Jordan in May 2001, he had to choose between peritoneal dialysis and hemodialysis. He chose the first option because he still worked five days a week and wanted to do the dialysis exchange himself every four hours. The advantage of peritoneal dialysis was that regular visits to a dialysis unit were not required. Martin needed surgery to place a catheter in his belly.

What we didn't know then is that bacteria entered the catheter and unfortunately this caused peritonitis several times. The doctor had mentioned a kidney-pancreas transplant as an option to increase the quality of his life, but if he had recurrent peritonitis this could be a problem. He advised him to switch to hemodialysis, and that meant another surgery to create vascular access in his arm, and three times a week on a dialysis machine for four hours in the hospital. On the days he was scheduled for dialysis treatment, Martin worked in the morning and went to the hospital in the afternoon. He drove himself until one day his shunt opened again after dialysis. While he was walking in the hallway of the hospital, he felt drops on his hand and when he looked, he saw the blood gushing out of his arm. He rushed to the dialysis unit, and thankfully they were able to help him. When he called me from the hospital and told me what had happened, I was worried. He still had to drive home, and all I could think of was: what if it happens again while he is driving? When Martin got home, he was covered in the blood that he lost in that short amount of time he walked from the dialysis unit to the hallway. I had already filled the bathtub with cold water and soaked his jacket and shirt in it. This is a perfect way to get blood out of clothes. The water turned red immediately and as I'm writing this, I can smell the blood again. Since that day we decided that I would pick him up after dialysis because both of us found it too risky if this would happen while he was driving. Not only that, but Martin also often felt too sick to drive. So besides having a full-time job, I was also the driver, the cook, the cleaner, the groceries woman, and the caregiver of my loved one. Yes, caregiving is hard.

What I didn't know about caregiving is that I would have less than eight hours of sleep a night. I had a lack of sleep, lived in fear, and felt alone sometimes. I remember one night when Martin's blood sugar was low. He had switched from long-acting insulin to short-acting insulin, and this was a complete disaster. I guess because we are so connected, I always woke up before him. That night I woke up at 1 AM because he was restless and mumbling in his sleep. I knew that he was having a hypoglycemic reaction and went downstairs to get some Extran (energy drink) and a small sugar sachet. Extran always helped Martin raise his blood sugar level quickly. Unfortunately, that night he refused to drink, and I tried the sugar. I stayed calm and talked slowly:

"Martin, could you do me a favor and take this sugar?"

"Yeah sure" with his eyes still closed.

Before I could put the sugar in his mouth, he waved his hands, and the content of the sugar sachet was all over the bed. I counted to ten because I was mad. Not at him, but the disease. I didn't have time to stay mad because raising his blood sugar was a top priority. Even though I knew I had to clean the bed afterward, I tried to stay calm and talked slowly again:

"Martin, if you drink the Extran, you will feel much better, and we can go to sleep after I have changed the bed. Ok?"

"Yeah sure." And thankfully he drank some of the Extran. After a few minutes, he opened his eyes and asked:

"What happened, what's in the bed. Is this sugar?" He looked at me and knew what had happened and felt sorry for me. I cleaned the bed, vacuumed and we went to sleep; I had to get up at 5.30 AM to go to work. Martin had many hypoglycemic episodes but thankfully he was conscious nine of the ten times. We always had Extran and food with us when we were on the road; just in case his blood sugar got too low.

> *Dear Caregiver,*
> *Do you sometimes get angry? If so, are you angry at the person or the disease and how do you deal with it?*

Diabetes is a nasty illness, and unfortunately, it has caused neuropathy for Martin. The nerves in his foot are damaged and he can walk with a pin in his foot without feeling anything. That's why he isn't allowed to walk with bare feet. Martin broke his ankle on July 7, 2009, while playing football with my nephews in the park. He didn't notice it because of the neuropathy. We thought his ankle was sprained. I was concerned about his ankle still being swollen after one week, and we went to see the doctor in the hospital. He had to stay the night, and an x-ray showed that he had a fracture on the left side of his left ankle. He had a cast for almost eight weeks and the fracture healed. We had planned a Panama Canal cruise in September to celebrate our 4th wedding anniversary. But Martin's ankle was still swollen, and we thought that it was because of the healing process of the fracture. Since we didn't trust it, we went to see the doctor again in the hospital.

"I'm sorry, but you have to cancel the cruise! Martin needs surgery."

Martin had taken a wrong step and broke the lateral malleolus bone of his ankle. We just don't know when this happened. He had surgery and a cast for another six to eight weeks. During that time, I was working, the driver, cook, cleaner, caregiver again. But that's not all! When the cast came off, we saw that Martin's ankle had grown crooked. After many appointments and x-rays, they found out that the surgery didn't go as planned. They hung the bone too high and that's why his ankle grew crooked. Martin made more bone but at the wrong place: on top of his ankle bone.

Another time of appointments, anger, and disappointment arose. Martin didn't fit in his shoes anymore and needed orthopedic shoes. These shoes had to be adjusted at least twenty times. Accepting the fact that he couldn't wear his modern shoes anymore, and the constant pain in his foot wasn't doing his mood any good. Not only that, but Martin also started having an ulcer under his foot, and because of the neuropathy we found out too late. At a certain point, the ulcer was almost an inch deep. In the hospital, they removed calluses many times, but that didn't help because the nasty stuff was underneath. He even had a cast for six weeks, but that didn't help either. The ulcer was very deep, all the way up to his bone. One day I went into the treatment room with Martin and watched the nurse clean the ulcer. Blood and pus were coming out of it.

"Are you ok Meriam?"

"Yes, I am."

Then she took a syringe and filled it with disinfectant and went into the ulcer. I can imagine if you feel nauseous right now.

Yes, we caregivers go through a lot. During the procedure, Martin was having a conversation with the nurse, because he didn't feel any pain. I told you: diabetes is a nasty illness! Note that this procedure was done without anesthesia. As I was watching this all very closely many things went through my mind. I was the one who should do this at home three times a day. Doing it myself would save me driving back and forth to the hospital daily. I asked the nurse for help; I needed to know how to clean the ulcer, I needed sterilized syringes, compresses, band-aids, tweezers, and all other medical supplies. Martin used crutches for weeks, and I cleaned the ulcer every single day, and we could go for a check-up every four or five days. Within a couple of weeks, it was healed, but we still had to be careful and check his foot daily. It happened a couple of times that we noticed an ulcer too late, but as soon as I started the cleaning procedure it healed within a few days.

One year later, in September 2010, we went on the Panama Canal cruise and celebrated another victory. Yes, Martin needed extra care, accepted the orthopedic shoes, and this will be the same for the rest of his life. Because his ankle is crooked, we have to stay on top of any hidden ulcers under his foot. But we won't let this dominate our lives.

Dear Caregiver,
Do you clean your loved ones' wounds, and do you ask medical professionals for help if you're stuck?

What if… what if…what if…

What if something happens when I leave him alone? I asked myself this question many times. Especially when he had hypoglycemic episodes daily. What if something happened to him while I was running errands, having a drink with a friend, at work or when he was on his way to work. I called Martin often to check on him and that didn't work. We were making ourselves crazy. I was restless, got tired, and exhausted. FEAR is a KILLER!

Martin had acupuncture treatments every week, and that helped him a bit. The guy who was treating Martin was a tall Dutch guy who was working closely together with Chinese alternative doctors. According to these doctors, this Dutch guy was the acupuncture guru. He knew a Chinese herbal doctor who had Qi-Kong classes every week. One day when he was treating Martin, he looked at me and said:

"I can tell that you are tired Meriam. Why don't you and Martin try the Qi-Kong classes? It could help both of you boost your energy. And it can also be considered a self-care moment."

"I don't have time for that" was my first reaction.

"You don't have time for your well-being?" he asked. "You are suffering from sleep deprivation; you are tired Meriam. I think that both of you can benefit from those classes. Why don't you give it a try?"

Martin was eager to start and suggested that we should try the classes.

"What if this does help and makes me feel better?" I thought. I flipped the negative "what if".

We arranged a consultation with the Chinese herbal doctor and decided to start with the 1-hour classes that started at 7 PM. I will never forget the first lesson. We were in a group of six or seven people. When everybody introduced themselves, he explained what we could feel while doing the exercises and I thought: ok this is a piece of cake; let's do this!

We started doing very slow movements with the arms.

"Is this it? Man, I can do this for hours."

After a few minutes, I felt tingling in my fingers and that was normal, he said. After doing the exercises for 15 minutes, I felt like I had been spinning for an hour. Wow, I never thought that those slow movements could have such an effect. That hour of Qi-Kong boosted my energy. Martin remembers his first session as if it was yesterday. He arrived there in a bad physical and mentally tired condition and left revitalized. That night, for the first time in months, both of us slept like a baby. Eight hours straight!

We went to the classes every week, and besides being a Chinese herbal doctor and Qi-Kong trainer, he was also a Reiki master. Martin had a weekly consult with him and was provided with herbs. I remember the first time when Martin went to the toilet after he drank his first herbal tea; that smell was awful. I noticed that after weeks of acupuncture, Reiki treatments, drinking herbal tea, and the Qi-Kong classes, Martin was feeling better even though he was on dialysis.

His blood sugar was stable, and my fear was decreasing. Our Reiki master told me more than once that I could help Martin too and taught me how and where to put my hands on Martin's body to transfer energy. When I did this, the middle of my hands got warm, and Martin could feel the energy. The idea that I was helping him made me feel good. After a couple of weeks, our Reiki master asked us both if we wanted to be initiated to Reiki 1 and we said yes. This all happened in early 2003.

I still help Martin when he needs some energy, and I can do this when I am in a space of love and not fear. As you know I was in fear earlier and the "what if" crossed my mind many times; it created negative thoughts. This exhausted me, lowered my energy, and made me feel sad.

But I flipped the negative thought into a positive thought by saying: "what if it all goes well?

I felt better when thinking of the outcome I desired or could imagine. And as soon as the "yeah, but.." came to my mind, I skipped the "but" and kept the "yeah." So it was: "Yeah, what if it all goes well?"

When you are in fear, please remember this mindset trick. It took me months to practice this, but I kept trying. One practice I adopted was doing Qi-Kong and focusing on my breathing and meditation.

The result of this was that I slept better. I was feeling more relaxed even though caregiving was tough. Making time to go to the Qi-Kong classes was a good decision; I am grateful that both Martin and I enjoyed the practice of self-care. Of course, he had days when he was feeling terrible, and I had to do more as his caregiver, but I was happy I took the opportunity to fill my cup so I could help him from my overflow.

After practicing Qi-Kong for a couple of months, we heard that Martin was number one on the transplant list. This was great news, and we were excited by the idea that the quality of both our lives would increase. But sometimes I felt alone; why me, why Meriam.

I was not alone; there was enough support from family and friends who asked me how I was doing, or if I needed help. My answer was that I was ok, but that was a lie. Pride was getting in the way of help sometimes. Especially when I had my super-shero cape on.

Super-sheroes don't need help, they can do it all by themselves.

I didn't do self-care in the beginning because I always thought that I had no time. But the thing is: I had to make time! There were lots of times when I felt alone because I was standing in my way. It took me years and a burnout to wake up and realize that I was not alone.

People reached out to me, but I thought I could do caregiving alone, and because I thought so I ended up feeling alone.

Dear Caregiver,
Do you feel this way sometimes?

And that's why communication is so important. I remember that I used to worry about what others might think of me. Why don't they get me? Don't they understand that caregiving is an exhausting job? Can't they see that I don't have time to go out for a drink?

One day at the office I talked to a colleague.

"Meriam, you're yawning so often, did you have a good night's rest?"

"No, I did not."

"How come?"

I looked at her and had to count to twenty before I gave my answer. Doesn't she get it? She knows I am a caregiver, why does she ask me this!

I decided to explain why I did not sleep well and told her my story. After five minutes I saw the tears in her eyes.

"Sorry, I knew you were a caregiver, but I had no idea it was this hard."

"No, thank you! Because of you, I realize that I should communicate better so others can get me."

Too often we think about what others might think or not. What if it all goes well when we tell them how and what we go through? When we don't ask for help, sometimes we exclude the people who want to help us the most. Even when we don't mean to.

In the beginning, when Martin was suffering from kidney failure, I didn't ask my mom-in-law for help. The reason I didn't do it is because of her age. And now I realize that I was overthinking. I should have asked her so she could decide if and when she was able to offer help or not. As a mother, she would always help her child when needed. Not only that, but she could also be part of her son's recovery.

There was a time when I had to leave Martin for one week to take care of myself (you will read more about this later). My mom-in-law took care of him, together with the rest of the family. I always enjoy the moments when I see her with Martin. She's 96 years old now but has a young spirit. Uses her iPhone and iPad, and is texting, face timing, and sending emails to her loved ones. I wish I had asked her for help more often. Know that I don't feel guilty about not doing so, but I just want to make it clear that asking for help also requires communication and no overthinking. All three of us won when I left for one week: Martin was taken care of, I could take care of myself, and she had quality time with her son.

Dear Caregiver,
Do you ask your in-laws for help?

In the spring of 2003, the doctor told Martin that he was number one on the transplant list. We had to be stand-by; we should be able to be in the hospital within one hour if they called. At that time, I had left the tax lawyer's office and was working for the government.

On November 23, 2003, at 10.15 AM, I received a phone call from the head of the dialysis department that he couldn't reach Martin. It was time!! Time for the kidney-pancreas transplant surgery. I couldn't believe my ears and didn't say a word for five seconds.

"Meriam, are you still there?"

"Yes, I'll try to reach Martin, and tell him to come to the hospital right away for his dialysis treatment."

What I didn't know is that Martin was in a meeting and had left his mobile phone on his desk. I kept calling and after fifteen minutes he returned my call and I told him: "it's time!"

Martin didn't quite understand me and said: "time for what dear?"

"Time for our new life! You can get a kidney-pancreas transplant surgery today honey."

Martin was quiet, and after a few seconds he said: "ok, I'll go to the hospital as soon as possible."

Martin had to do a dialysis treatment first in the hospital where he always went, but the surgery would be done in another hospital. But there was a but..! Everything should be 100% ok with both Martin and the organs. The nephrologist had to run some tests while he was on dialysis, and he wasn't allowed to eat or drink anything from the moment he received the phone call.

I went home by public transport, packed his bag with clothes and toiletries, took the car, and went to the hospital. When I arrived there, Martin had already started his dialysis treatment. He had to be "clean" before surgery. I called his mom to tell her that it was time for her son to get the transplant surgery and she came to the hospital as soon as she could. In the meantime, the doctors of both hospitals connected. It was 3:30 PM when the doctor of the dialysis department came into the room and said:

"All the test results are perfect. Martin can go. Please drive as quickly as you can to the ER of the other hospital."

We were right in time before the traffic jams and the ER crew of the other hospital was already waiting for us. We were escorted to the transplant unit. Martin was very hungry, but that poor guy wasn't allowed to eat or drink anything. The anesthesiologist and surgeon came into the room and told us that the organs were on their way. I imagined a cool box with ice and two organs in a plastic bag. The organs should be checked again, and they had to do some more tests. If there was one single thing that wasn't okay, the surgery would be canceled at the very last minute. Imagine that you have been waiting for this moment for years, preparing for surgery since early morning, hoping to start a new chapter in your life and you hear in the evening that the moment you've been waiting for is canceled. I didn't give this negative thought a chance to stay in mind and flipped it: what if it all goes well and he has surgery tonight!

I started praying. It was 8 PM. Still nothing…No news from the doctors yes.. At 8.20 PM the nurse came to us and said:

"BINGO! Martin, you are ready for the OR."

Within ten minutes the nurses took care of everything, and my mom-in-law and I brought Martin as far as allowed before he went to the OR. The surgeon told us that surgery could take between six to nine hours and asked me if I wanted to stay in the hospital, but I chose to go home with my mom-in-law. I wanted to be in my environment. The surgeon promised me that he would call me after he was done with Martin. My mom-in-law and I were tired of all that had happened earlier and went to bed around 10:30 PM.

I woke up at 3 AM and started praying that the surgery would go well and that Martin would have a speedy recovery. At 3:15 AM the phone rang, and I recognized the phone number: it was the surgeon. I waited for a few seconds before I answered with a dry mouth.

"Meriam speaking."

I heard the surgeon's voice saying: "Meriam, we are done with surgery. Everything went very well. I have never transplanted such beautiful organs. Martin is doing fine."

Once I heard this, tears began to roll down my face. And as I'm writing this my eyes are filled with tears. Tears of joy!

You see, we had been waiting for this moment for years. Especially Martin, who has been a diabetic as of his 15th, suffering from kidney failure and being on dialysis. Having a kidney-pancreas transplant was the chance to improve the quality of his life. I asked the surgeon what time I could visit Martin, and he said that any time after 8 AM was ok, but that I shouldn't be afraid when I saw him. There would be a lot of beeping of medical devices he was connected to.

I hung up and went to my mom-in-law's bedroom. When I opened the door, she could see the relief and happiness on my face. We embraced and didn't speak; we just held each other. I could feel her heart just pounding against mine as her tears wet my shoulder. I was so happy I was not alone at that moment.

After a few minutes, we dried our tears and started smiling. We still didn't say a word; we just hugged again, and I told her we should get some more sleep and that we could see him later.

> *Dear Caregiver,*
> *Have you ever communicated without words?*

A few hours later, around 7 AM, I woke up and prepared an email for family and friends to inform them that Martin went into surgery the night before and that it all went well. At 10 AM, my mom-in-law and I went to the ICU to visit him.

When we arrived in the room, he was still connected to many medical devices. He was sleeping, and when I whispered his name, he opened one eye and smiled. I kissed him on his cheek, and I couldn't stop looking at the healthy color on his face. I held his hand, and I said:

"Honey, we did it."

He was still groggy because of the drugs, but he managed to open both his eyes, smiled at me, and said:

"Yes, we did it."

His mom kissed him on his forehead and said:

"I am so proud of you son."

Martin had a scar from his chest up to under his navel. It looked like a zipper because of the staples they used to close the wound. We only stayed for only a couple of minutes and went to the restaurant for a cup of coffee. Both of us were captured in our thoughts and didn't talk for a few minutes. I felt like all the tension of waiting years for this moment was fading away slowly. Although I was tired and sleepy, I felt relief and happiness. We did it!

I was grateful that Martin had a second chance. We never lost hope and yes: Chapter 2.0 had begun!

But how will he recover? This question still crossed my mind.

Weeks went by and even though I was happy that Martin had his first kidney-pancreas transplant surgery I was still running the whole day. While he was recovering from surgery, I had to take care of many other things besides my full-time job. Let me give you an idea of what my day looked like.

I woke up at 5:30 AM and started between 7 – 7:30 AM at the office. After work, I went home by public transport, took the car, and drove for fifty minutes to the hospital. I stayed there until 9 – 9:30 PM, so Martin and I could have dinner together. When I was home around 10 – 10:15 PM, I checked emails, did household chores or watched tv, and fell asleep around midnight or later.

This was my routine for many weeks. This exhausted me, but I kept going. Unfortunately, I didn't attend the Qi-Kong classes anymore; I was not taking good care of myself.

And it wasn't until a social worker asked me in a conversation with her and Martin: "Meriam, how are you doing?"

My world fell apart, and for fifteen minutes, I cried and sobbed like a child. I was so mad at this social worker for asking me this question; for making me cry in front of Martin. I didn't want him to see me like this; I was the super-shero who could do the caregiving by herself. But I thought wrong, and I had burnt out!

We caregivers sometimes ignore the signs of our body when it says: I need a timeout! Our plate might get too full when we take care of others. It's not done on purpose; it happens because we care and want to offer our help. The question of why this is happening to us might come to our minds, and at the same time, we wonder if there are possibilities to be productive while taking care of our loved ones.

> *Dear Caregiver:*
> *Have you ever felt like you just want to breathe for a couple of minutes? Or how you can make time to have some me-time?*

You see, the question of the social worker saved my life. When I came home, I looked in the mirror and said:

"Meriam, what are you going to do for you?" To be honest, I couldn't answer. I looked in the mirror again and said:

"Meriam, what-are-you-going-to-do-for-you? What if something happens to you? Who's going to take care of Martin? Name one good reason why you ignore the signs of your body. Just one!"

I could NOT answer.

This was my wake-up call. I felt awful, sick, and I knew I had to do something about it, otherwise, it could have a bad effect on both our lives. I needed time to find out how to breathe, and when to do self-care, how to ask for help, and more. Martin was still recovering from the major surgery, but I needed a break. The next day, Martin and I talked about what had happened, and it was a wake-up call for him as well.

I decided to leave for one week and asked my mom-in-law to be with her son and of course she was more than willing to help. I went to Surinam, and I have to tell you that I did NOT feel guilty. It was a difficult decision but the best thing I could do at that time. Going on a break while your husband is in the hospital is heartbreaking, but it was either that or my health would go wrong.

When I left, I had to work on myself and learn how to revitalize my energy. The exhaustion was beyond words. I didn't know where to start. But I had been going for too long and ignoring the unwanted feelings. Caregivers often don't show their emotions. We sometimes act like super-sheroes who don't get sick and think that we can do it all by ourselves. If something happened to me, who would take care of Martin?

We cannot expect the people we are caregiving for to notice we may be close to burnout. We are the only ones who can take care of ourselves.

Dear Caregiver,
I ask that you take care of yourself.

After I came back from Surinam, Martin was losing too much weight. At first, they connected the pancreas to the urinary bladder but somehow Martin's body discharged all the salt. At a certain point, he had to take more than fifty salt pills a day. In those days, they waited for twelve months to do the second surgery to connect the pancreas to the small intestine. But in Martin's case, they had to do it three months after the first surgery. And even though the fear and "what if" took a new seat in my mind, I never lost hope. Fortunately, things went well after the second surgery in February 2004, and Martin gained weight very quickly. I was still beating my burnout and for the first time, I dared to think about having a small holiday break and started looking for possibilities. Yes, we deserved the first break after a time of living in fear, with exhaustion and burnout. We decided to drive to Bruges, Belgium, and enjoyed four days in a small family hotel in April 2004.

It felt unreal, no dialysis, no insulin needed, eating whenever he wanted, drinking as much as he wanted, it was unreal…

Everything went well since his second surgery, although Martin had several other surgeries (both eyes and ankle). But the quality of his life went from 2 to 8.

What I learned the most from this experience is that BELIEF is crucial. I ASKED for strength for both of us and we RECEIVED it to cope with the situation.

Dear Caregiver,
Do you ASK for help and if so, how and when?

Martin and I had been to Surinam when he was on peritoneal dialysis, and we stayed at mom's place. She enjoyed every moment we spent together. I don't regret the many times I went alone to Surinam when Martin was doing much better. Mom was getting older and was suffering from high blood pressure and had a minor cerebral hemorrhage a couple of times. My oldest sister and niece took care of her and when I was there, they could get some relief and take care of themselves more often.

Dear Caregiver,
Do you ask your siblings or other family members to help take care of your parents?

Early April 2011, I received a phone call from my oldest sister. Mom was in the hospital; she had a severe cerebral hemorrhage and was not doing well. I purchased a ticket to Surinam and on Monday, April 11, 2011, I called my sister when she and my niece were visiting mom, who didn't talk anymore. I asked my niece to hold the phone next to mom's ear so she could hear me. As I told mom that I would be there next Friday, I could hear her breathing. She gathered all her energy and said: yes! I had hope, but I couldn't explain why I was still feeling sad.

The next morning while I was in a meeting with the team my phone rang. It was Patrick saying: "mom left us Meriam". I looked at my supervisor whom I had told that my mom was in a critical condition, and she could tell by the look in my eyes that mom had gained her wings. The tears started rolling over my cheeks and the question "WHY?" came into my head. "Why didn't you wait for me mom?". My world fell apart, my heart broke into a thousand pieces. Why didn't she wait for me? A couple of hours ago she said "yes!" when I told her I was coming to take care of her.

Within a few days, the whole family went to Surinam. Mom always told us that she wanted to be cremated and that she wanted to wear her purple dress and hat. This clever woman wanted to leave earth like a queen. We never wanted to talk about her death, but she insisted.

"It's part of life, my child. You will thank me later."

And yes, we thanked her. We only had to carry out her assignment and didn't have to think about what she would have wanted after she had gone to rest. Mom was a beloved woman, and many people called us before the cremation to ask if they could send flowers. We asked for a donation, even though we didn't know yet what we would do with it.

Mom was cremated seven days after she died. Approximately three hundred people showed their respect and two days later we threw her ashes in the river;

just as she wished. The same river of the district where she was born, had grown up, and her dad had brought kids to school. Later that day, all of us were sitting on the porch, and I asked the family if anybody had an idea what we could do with the huge amount of money people donated. My niece, daughter of my late sister, who was living with mom and took care of her, came up with a brilliant idea.

"Why don't we help a kid's shelter?"

"Which one?" I asked.

"Well, there is a woman who's taking care of children with HIV between the ages of two to eighteen years. She doesn't have any subsidy from the government and depends on donations and volunteers to help her with taking care of the kids."

None of us had to think twice and we were so excited about this idea. The next day we called the kids shelter and asked the founder what they needed. Together with my niece and her four-year-old daughter I went to the supermarket and bought everything that was asked. When we arrived at the shelter, we met the founder. The children just came back from a 1-day excursion, and you could tell they had a great time. The founder was very happy with all the things we brought, but she was also curious why we did it. My niece told her that her grandmother loved children, and when she died people wanted to send flowers, but we asked for a donation instead. With that money, we bought all she had asked for and we knew that mom would be thrilled with this idea.

The founder's eyes filled with tears, and she couldn't stop thanking us. It felt so good: even if you are in grief, you can make others happy!

This shelter took care of those kids with HIV and this aligned with what mom did in her life. Both were caregivers. This was a nice gesture. From a late caregiver to a caregiver who was doing her best to let those kids feel loved, forget their illness for a while by taking them on a break, teach them how to deal with their illness, and let them know they were not alone.

I know mom would love this idea; somehow the atmosphere in the shelter reminded me of the day mom took care of me when I was a seven-year-old child with a fever. How she had beaten the fever with the herbs in the calabash. The love and the idea that there was someone who took care of me made me feel good. Thank you, mom!

Dear Caregiver,
Do you talk about death with your loved one?

Martin had to arrange a flight to Surinam for the cremation, but all the straight flights were fully booked. The only option for him was to fly via Curacao but then he had to stay one night on the island. Thankfully my BFF took good care of him. Martin arrived just in time for the cremation. I was able to change my flight from Surinam, so we could fly home together via Curacao after the cremation.

Leaving Surinam after mom's death was heavy on the heart. Both my parents were gone and saying goodbye to my family wasn't easy. I remember my BFF, her sister, and brother-in-law picking us up at the airport. When I saw my BFF, I started crying without even saying a word. I was sobbing and her sister and brother-in-law came and hugged us. It was a group hug, and no one was saying anything. Grief, sadness, pain; they could feel all my emotions. We went home and I took a shower, and when we all sat on the porch, I told them what had happened; how it all went, and how I felt not having parents anymore. The boys of my BFF who were six and seven years old at that time also comforted me and that was so sweet. The youngest boy is my godson. I could let my tears flow without feeling silly. They knew auntie just lost her mom and that she was very sad.

My BFF and I talked for hours, till late at night. This time we had serious conversations about our lives, the circle of life, the lessons we learned, and the goals we wanted to achieve. She was there for me; listening to me, comforting me, holding me. And I listened to her; how she was doing as an unexpected widow and mom who worked full-time. Two years earlier her husband died after they had been living on the island for only three months.

We filled each other's cup; again! Like we have been doing for the last thirty-five years.

After a couple of days of spending time with the family in Curacao, Martin and I left; knowing we would be back soon. My BFF, her boys, sister, and brother-in-law took care of me while I was there with Martin. I felt heard, I felt loved, I wasn't alone, and the feeling that I, caregiver Meriam, was taken care of gave me the power to move forward.

Dear Caregiver,
Do you have someone you can talk to?

My BFF's brother-in-law would turn 50 in September 2011 and there was a party planned. Martin and I went back to Curacao; it always felt like going home. We usually rented a car, so we could get groceries, pick the boys up from school, or have lunch with my BFF. There was a nice restaurant close to her office, and we always ordered her food before she arrived, so we could enjoy lunch together.

Martin was feeling much better and also enjoyed helping my BFF with things that should be done in and around the house. Her brother-in-law's birthday party was a blast! Imagine a house on a hill with a pool and an AH-MA-ZING view from the porch. All was taken care of, and everything happened around the pool: there was a live band, a bar with delicious cocktails, and a buffet. My BFF enjoyed every minute with her parents and family. It brings a smile to my face when I think of those moments.

My BFF and I got used to seeing each other at least once or twice a year. Taking care of each other was necessary. I have been to Curacao many times and always enjoyed the temperature, the atmosphere, the family: yes, that's what my BFF and loved ones are. The moments I spent there and the conversations I had with my BFF are priceless. Curacao gave me a lot in many ways: physically because whenever I was there, I could rest, have me-time, even if it sometimes meant watching an iguana from the porch having breakfast, and mentally because I could reset and charge my battery for when I got back home in the Netherlands.

And so, until 2014, we went to Curacao as often as we could. In the summer of that year, my BFF moved back to the Netherlands. Instead of nine hours flying, the distance between us is only one hour driving now. We plan a spa day once or twice a year; just the two of us. On this day we are revitalizing our energy, talking, laughing, and of course, we ask each other for help if needed.

When I ask for help, I always explain to the person I'm asking why I'm asking. Clarity is important and so is communication. I also inform the person that it is ok if what I'm asking for can't be done.

Asking for help means that if I get help, I get relief for a moment because I don't have to do something myself. The relief means that I can breathe, that I can have me-time.

And me-time means that I can do self-care.

> *Dear Caregiver,*
> *Do you think it feels weird to ask for help in the beginning?*

Asking for help is a practice and commitment because we sometimes don't want to ask for help. The question is why? I bet that when someone asks you for something you will do it if you can. Why is it ok for you to give and not ok to receive? I practiced asking for help every day.

"Can you help me with cleaning the windows?"

"Can you drive me to the hospital next Saturday?"

"Can you help me get groceries?"

"Can you stay with Martin so I can go get a massage?"

I was amazed to see how people were willing to help. I even asked my neighbors for help. I was committed to keeping asking for help because it took away the feeling of being alone and it gave me time for myself. I have to be honest that in the beginning, it felt weird.

"Why would you ask them to help you? They have a busy schedule too!"

There was that negative chatter again and sometimes it won, and I ended up not asking for help.

Result: I got exhausted. And that's exactly what I didn't want. I had to take action and Ask for Help!

It took a lot of courage to ask for help because I was more willing to give than to receive. Yes, read that again. I felt more comfortable when I helped others, and I thought I didn't need help from others. I thought of what people would think of me or that they would think that I was weak and that I couldn't handle caregiving.

Today I think that NOT asking for help was a sign of my weakness! Today I can stand in my power because I get help and thus relief. Please, stop asking yourself the question of what others will think of you if you ask for help. Stop thinking "what if..". Stop feeling guilty when you ask for help so you can breathe.

When you care for your loved one you feel like you help someone get through the day, you feel gratitude. When Patrick was showered and dressed in the hospital I was tired, but he felt clean and refreshed. The smile on his face was priceless.

Caregiving drains us because we don't make and take the time to breathe. I started owning my well-being by doing ten to fifteen minutes of breathing exercises per day or doing something else I love. Sometimes I just did nothing. I was more focused on myself but before I could do this as a caregiver, I needed to ask for help.

We sometimes are too focused on the question: "what will other people think of me when…" "what if.."

Before we even know it, we are only focused on our loved ones instead of ourselves.

> *So dear Caregiver,*
> *I'm curious: how do you ask for help? Do you just pop the question, or do you think for at least an hour before you ask someone for help? How do you ask for help?*

Many of us don't have a problem with giving, we have a problem with receiving. When I needed help, I had at least two people in mind that I could ask for help for the same thing. I always had a backup! If the one wasn't able to help, I still had another person who I could ask for help.

Here's a small tip that might help you. Check your list of contacts on your phone and decide who is good at cooking, cleaning etcetera. Create your list of helpers. A sort of an emergency caregivers list. Remember I told you to check for possibilities?

Sometimes it's still hard for me to ask for help. Especially when I think that it's an easy job that I can do myself, but I KNOW it will stress me out because my schedule will be too tight. This happens when the little voice, that little negative chatter in my head says:

"Meriam, don't be silly to ask for help, you can do this. Just squeeze it in between the two other tasks on your "to-do" list."

Yes, this nasty chatter will always be in the background, but I now know how to deal with it.

Congratulations! You have started to strengthen the A of your Personal Assistant SOS with an extra S (PASOSS).

Keep FOLLOW in mind:

Forgive yourself

Be **O**pen-minded

Listen to your gut

Learn new things

See and grab **O**pportunities

Know your **W**orth

SCHEDULING AND ORGANIZING

I recognized that when you are a caregiver your time is determined by your loved one's appointments, showering, or the meals that need to be made. There might be so many external requirements that mark your schedule.

The question I asked myself is: what do I value about myself, and my loved one, what do I value about time to come up with that schedule. And what happens if I see a day, week, or month differently.

Something that helped me was renaming my recurring tasks in my calendar e.g. preparing dinner. I named it "preparing the boost of our energy."

Working out was: "making sure I fit in that beautiful lace dress.". Now I would add a dress emoji to my digital calendar. If I rename my tasks, I'm more likely to do it because of the positive tweak I've given to them.

Another thing I would like to add is that if you schedule something for yourself, some me-time, or another positive thing might come out of it. Positivity creates possibility.

Let me give you an example. After Martin's second surgery, I was still coping with my burnout. But I was too determined for us both to have some me-time, and I scheduled a 4-day break to Bruges, Belgium. This was our first holiday in a long time and yes, we were both excited, but also a bit nervous. But when we discovered how much ease and relief this short getaway gave us, we wanted to schedule a new retreat. The "what if his body rejects the organs" faded away slowly, and in February 2005 we took a 10-hour flight to Miami to go on our first Caribbean Cruise. We were able to see more possibilities within our situation.

If you rethink your scheduling, that tells the universe that you're open to other possibilities. If you had said to me in 2003 after Martin's first kidney-pancreas transplant surgery that within two years we would enjoy a Caribbean cruise, I would have said that it's impossible. Because I would have to figure out how and what the medical staff could do onboard a ship, or if there were transplant specialists in Miami.

If I hadn't scheduled a holiday break as in a cruise for us, I wouldn't have known that the ocean breeze calms me and revitalizes my energy. What I want to say is that don't underestimate the impact of scheduling. Once you do it, you might move something from the back to the front of the list, and the result of doing this can open possibilities for you.

You can create possibilities for both you, and your loved one by scheduling.

Dear Caregiver,

Are you feeling crazy because of all the things you have to remember? Are all appointments including doctor appointments on a sticky note on your fridge? Have you forgotten appointments and been charged for them? And has all of that drained you? And so, are you stuck and feel guilty when you've forgotten an appointment? Or caregiver, have you overscheduled and forgotten yourself? Are you on your to-do list and prioritizing yourself?

Yes, caregiver, I do have a lot of questions for you. For those of you who are struggling with scheduling: know that it will clear your head. It will also give you an overview, and the opportunity to make time for yourself. Yes, read the last four words again!

I remember a day when I was at the office, and I received a phone call from the hospital.

"Hello?"

"Hi, is this Meriam? Sister of Patrick?"

"Yes, speaking."

"Oh ok great: We are waiting for Patrick."

"When? Now?"

"Yes, Patrick has an appointment today."

My mind was racing. I was searching for this appointment in my head but couldn't find it.

"Hello, are you still there?"

"Uhm , yes. I think I forgot the appointment."

"Ok, we can reschedule, but please know that we have to charge you for this one."

"Yeah, I understand."

But I lied; I did not understand. My brother would be charged for not showing up because I forgot the appointment. How could I forget it? It was too important to miss such an appointment, and I wanted to ask the doctor some questions. I felt guilty. I should have known better because since my burnout I started scheduling. I remember that my brother received a letter with a date and time for his doctor's appointment, and I didn't put it in my calendar right away. I thought that when I was home I could do it. And that's where it went wrong.

Dear Caregiver,
Have you ever missed an appointment because you kept it all in your mind? And has it cost you money?

I called my brother and explained what had happened and that I would pay the bill. I could have had a nice dinner for that amount and the more I thought about it, the more I felt miserable. Scheduling would have saved me from having these frustrating feelings. But I forgave myself and I was reminded why it is so important to schedule.

Do you know who was a good scheduler? My grandpa, mom's dad! He scheduled without a computer, phone, tablet, or any other fancy device. At forty years old, he became a caregiver after his wife died at the age of thirty-five. While grieving, he took care of his five young children. He scheduled and organized: the oldest girl cooked and helped with taking care of the two-year-old while he was away. The boys who were eight and eleven years old helped with cleaning the yard and planting vegetables. In those days the women took care of the household, and the men worked on the field. Grandpa kept going and made sure his kids had no lack of love, food, and a roof above their heads. Imagine a two-year-old girl calling for her mom in the night. He made sure she was comforted when in need of her mom.

I was only seven years old when he died, and I was too young then to understand what he did to cope with the illness and loss of a loved one and taking care of five children. Now that I think back, I realize what he did.

Grandpa was a handsome tall skinny black man. He was fond of his children and grandchildren, and lived in a district, approximately thirty miles from the capital of Surinam. He enjoyed music and played the saxophone and the church organ every Sunday. That was his self-care moment.

His words *if you can't do good, don't harm* are etched in all of our minds. One of his stories I still remember is that he brought children to school with the boat. There were no roads, so he picked up the kids at certain points and brought them to the school which was next to the river. He was committed that the young ones were educated and that they should at least finish primary school. My oldest sister sometimes went with him as a child to bring the children to school. Most of the kid's parents or grandparents were originally from India, and grandpa communicated with them in Hindi and Surinamese.

Grandpa lived in a small wooden house on stone blocks. The journey from our house to grandpa's house took forever. First, we had to take the bus to the center of Paramaribo, and then we had to switch to the bus to Saramacca, the district where grandpa lived. Imagine a bus, fully packed with people from the district who bought a lot of stuff in the capital. In those days there were only a few supermarkets in the district, so people came to Paramaribo to shop. But the journey with the bus was worth it.

When you were at grandpa's place, there was space and with this, I mean that the yard was huge and filled with fruit trees, vegetables, flowers. I will never forget the smell of food which was prepared on wood. The atmosphere was amazing and even though it was old-fashioned, I look back at a time with joy. Grandpa died on Christmas day 1977, and every Christmas I think of him and thank him for his wise lessons. He taught me to pray, be respectful, but accept no disrespect from others. The love he had for his kids and grandkids was beyond, and he always said that the relationship between us should be strong. Thank you so much, grandpa!

Another amazing scheduler was my grandma (dad's mom). She was a beautiful and very strong woman who raised fifteen children. Yes, fifteen children! I once asked her how she dealt with the daily tasks and raising fifteen children and her answer was:

"my darling, in those days things were different. You had a lot of kids and the older ones helped with raising the young ones. The boys helped with fishing, hunting, and cleaning the yard, and the older girls helped with cooking and household. I also asked my siblings for help."

Grandma was scheduling and organizing without an iPad, mobile phone, or calendar.

Grandma lived in a wooden house near a busy street in Paramaribo. She had a beautiful shepherd dog who was very protective of her. He meant the world to her; she even brushed his teeth. She loved baking cookies and her typical Surinamese cakes were so delicious. Whenever it was one of her children's or grandchildren's birthdays, she baked a cake or cookies for them as her gift.

I remember her telling me the story of my grandpa. He came from Austria, and unfortunately died very young when he was in his thirties. I don't remember how he ended up in Surinam, but he and grandma had six children. After he died grandma met a Chinese man and she had another nine kids. When it was grandma's birthday it was just her kids, grandkids, and great-grandkids. She was a very rich woman; when she died, she had eighty-one grandkids and twenty-seven great-grandkids.

Dear Caregiver,
Do you take care of your kids and/or grandkids?
If so, do you schedule, especially now with the pandemic?

It was hard for me to schedule after my burnout, because it consumed time. I simply didn't want to add something else to my already busy to-do list. My plate was full, and I couldn't see how scheduling could help me. It was easier to keep it all in my head. And it would consume too much of my time; something I didn't have as a caregiver, cook, cleaner, driver!

What I didn't realize is that my refusal to schedule would end up draining me more and keeping me from being as productive and effective as I could be.

The time I didn't schedule but should have was when Martin had so many doctor's appointments. Trying to live your life and having so many other things to do daily required scheduling. I kept all the appointments in my head, and I can tell you that it was not a success. It made me feel drained because my head was too full. I used to forget what I should ask the doctor.

Martin and I have always asked lots of questions to the medical professionals. The questions included "what is the percentage of his kidney functioning; do you know who to contact about the dialysis center in Torremolinos, Spain in case of emergency during our holiday."

I was always sitting with a notebook taking notes. And if I didn't understand what the doctor was saying I asked for clarification. Remember: the doctor has limited time per patient, and you want to get all the answers you need. I recommend that before you go to an appointment, write your questions on a piece of paper or even better; put them in your notes on your mobile phone. Otherwise, you might forget. You don't want to be guessing about questions when you're driving home. When I saw that this worked, I started doing it for all appointments and even questions I have for friends and family.

Scheduling is a practice and a commitment. Believe me: it will clear your head. You don't have to remember it all. I recommend that you use a paper calendar and start scheduling per week. If you know you have a doctor's appointment next month, write it down and put a memory in the digital calendar if you have one. Practice, practice practice!

The benefits of scheduling:

Relief:
I experience it as my friend who makes sure I do the things that need to be done for both me and my loved one.

Clarity:
When someone asks to go for a drink or something else, I just consult my schedule, and I know if I can say Yes or No. Scheduling means being organized. If it's in my calendar, that means that it is important!

When I schedule, I feel organized in my head. I don't have to remember all the doctor appointments, medication schedules, me-time moments, or breathing moments.

I am so used to schedule that it's in my DNA now. Like asking for help, or checking possibilities, it was hard for me to make scheduling a habit. I used a seven-day paper calendar, so I could schedule per day.

Now I use my phone and computer to schedule all my appointments. I suggest that you start with a paper calendar because you will see it in writing and it's more likely that you will follow the schedule.

I can hear you think: but HOW am I going to do this? Let me give you some tips:

- Make it A Friday (or another weekday) morning habit to schedule for the upcoming week.
- Take an extra 15 minutes to BREATHE after every appointment
- Include your habits/me-time in your schedule.
- Give your me-time a powerful name e.g. Beautiful nails for Meriam!
- Print your weekly schedule or take a photo of it so you always have it with you.
- Put an alarm on your phone to remind you of your breathing moments.

- If you have a recurring appointment in a couple of months, put it in your phone right away or your paper calendar.

- If you have questions for the doctor or another medical professional, write your questions on a piece of paper or in your notes on your phone before you see him/her and take notes.

Reminder: Scheduling will eat up fifteen to twenty minutes of your time but will save you from getting drained or forgetting appointments. It will create time for you and provide you with more choices.

Caregiver, I want to ask you to be optimistic and laser-focused on seeing possibilities, asking for help, and scheduling. Please use all the techniques. One is connected to the other. To get results, you have to use them together or at least two or three together.

Let me give you an example: if you are tired, ask yourself the question: why? Because I don't take care of myself. How come? I don't have, make or take time. Do you schedule and organize? No. Then start with it to create time for yourself. Do you ask for help? No, I'm the only one who takes care of my loved one. Is there a social worker or other professional you can talk to? Maybe hire a private nurse for two hours per week? Or can you get respite care?

Scheduling is one step towards self-love. Scheduling and organizing in combination with asking for help will lead to self-care. Self-care will lead to less stress.

Congratulations! You have started to strengthen the SO of your Personal Assistant SOS with an extra S (PASOSS).

Keep FOLLOW in mind.

Forgive yourself

Be **O**pen- minded

Listen to your gut

Learn new things

See and grab **O**pportunities

Know your **W**orth

SELF-CARE

I love how I easily connect with people.
I love looking in the mirror and admire my beauty, inside and out.
I love my imperfection.
I love ME.

Dear Caregiver,
Do you love yourself? If so, can you name two things you do
to show it within fifteen seconds?

I remember that when I met Martin my weight was around 63 kg/138 lbs. We often went out for dinner and I gained weight fast. One of the main reasons was that I didn't go to the gym anymore. I got comments like: "wow, you gained weight" "life is good huh, I can tell". I knew I had gained weight, but those comments made me feel uncomfortable and insecure. One day I was sad and asked Martin if he still loved me because my body had changed.

"You are still the same Meriam that I met and fell in love with. The same Meriam that has one sentence with both Surinamese and Dutch words. The same Meriam that sometimes needs to thank Mother Earth with her calabash and water. The same Meriam who dances to traditional music. So yes, your body has changed, but Meriam hasn't changed. If you don't feel comfortable in this body, do something about it, but you have to know that I love Meriam."

I was speechless; I could be ME. His answer was so powerful and it gave me the self-confidence boost that I needed. I started loving ME and appreciating every curve of my body.

Dear Caregiver,
Do you love your body? If not, are you willing to do something about it? Do you have a favorite part of your body?

My eyes are my favorite part of my body. They can see what is going on with me and the loved ones I am focused on. I love the shape of my eyes, and I squint a little. Sometimes my eyes tell what I feel, what I might think and that's not always good. I guess that you can see people's feelings if you look at their eyes. Love, anger, disappointment, pain, happiness.

Yes, I love my eyes and they sometimes create a self-care moment for me when I put on some eyeshadow, eyeliner, or mascara. This self-care moment only lasts for a couple of minutes, but I always enjoy it. When I look in the mirror, I'm reminded of my beauty. I am grateful for my eyes that saw Martin having a severe hypoglycemic reaction and because I saw it, I could react quickly and call the paramedics. I am also grateful for my eyes who allow me to see both Martin and Patrick feeling happy again. My eyes are the favorite part of my body that I use to enjoy self-care moments with.

But I also remember a time when I needed to take care of another part of my body and do self-care. I was thirteen years old. One morning I woke up and had such a pain in my right boob. I couldn't touch it; it hurt that much. I went to school but wearing the bra was hurting me. When I got home, I told mom that I had such a pain in my boob. She asked me if she could take a look and that was ok with me. My late sister also took a look and told mom to take me to the doctor. That's when I said:

"No, I will be fine. There's no need for our old doctor to look at my boob. I'll be fine."

Mom and my sister knew why I didn't want to go to the doctor. I had never experienced showing private parts to a stranger. Anyways, it hurt so much that I had no choice. Mom took me to the doctor, and I remember the air-conditioned room; it was freezing. Mom told him what was wrong with me, and the doctor asked me to show him. I was not afraid but the idea of showing my private part was embarrassing. The doctor knew it and told me that it was ok; he wanted to help as a medical professional, and the only way for him to do so was to examine my breast. He could tell that I was in pain, and he needed to take a look at it. After a couple of minutes of comforting me, I decided to do it. I had to lie down on a treatment bed, and he examined me. I didn't look at him and I shied away. Because it was so cold in the room my nipples hurt and I felt embarrassed. Minutes seemed like hours and the exam took forever.

When the doctor was done with me, he told me and mom that he felt a lump and wanted me to see another doctor in the hospital the next day. I immediately asked if that doctor was a man or a woman. When he told me that it was a man, I wanted to cry but I knew I had no choice. Again: it was too painful. The next day my dad drove me and mom to the hospital and I remember this doctor being very kind and comforting.

He was a tall Dutch man and explained everything he would do and what I could feel. The room was also air-conditioned, and I thought: ok here we go again with the embarrassment. The doctor examined the lump and told us that I had an inflamed mammary gland. I had to make sure that I kept my boob moist the rest of the day and night. He wanted to wait one more day to see what would happen. Two things could happen: the inflammation could be cleaned by my body, or it would get worse, and then a procedure would be needed. He wanted to see me the next day again. I remember his words: take care of yourself and you will be ok. I didn't sleep well that night and mom checked on me a couple of times during the night.

The next morning, I felt less pain and didn't know if it was just because I wanted to feel less pain or if it was the case. We went to the hospital and when I entered the doctor's room, I was so nervous that I could feel my heart bouncing in my throat. I noticed that I was not embarrassed as I was the first time. When he examined my boob, it didn't hurt as much as the day before. He nodded and told me and mom that there was no procedure needed. My body was taking care of the lump itself. I saw the relief on mom's face, and I was happy with the news as well. I was embarrassed at first, but both male doctors comforted me, and their caring helped too.

Dear Caregiver,
Do you remember a time when you were both embarrassed and had to do self-care in order to stay healthy?

Self-care is necessary and means doing something YOU love. It doesn't matter what you do, as long as it's something you enjoy. You will revitalize your energy and will experience ease. The result of ease is relaxation. When you're relaxed you can think better and be more productive. The result is that you can be a better caregiver and that's a win-win situation for both you and your loved one. Doing self-care means loving yourself and owning your well-being.

One day in spring 2012 my supervisor asked me:

"Meriam, when are you finally going to do something with your communication skills?" Since she asked me that question, I couldn't get it out of my head. Another question that stopped me in my tracks.

A few days later I had a Surinamese party to attend. And you should know that when Surinamese women go to a party, they don't show up in jeans! I am a size 16 and I couldn't find a nice dress in my size.

I got so angry and told Martin: "I AM DONE WITH THIS. I AM GOING TO START MY WEBSHOP WITH EXCLUSIVE PLUS-SIZE CLOTHING!"

What started as an idea, became a desire, and I started collecting information on how to start my own business. I went to free courses offered by the tax department and chamber of commerce. I had to show the world that every(body) is beautiful! I was determined to give women (more) self-confidence when needed, empower them to be and love themselves.

I collected lots of information and was almost ready to start with the webshop. On November 7, 2012, I was at the office when I received a phone call from Martin.

"You HAVE to call Patrick NOW!"

"What's wrong with him?"

"I don't have time to explain dear, but please call him immediately. He just called me, and I think there's something wrong with him. He was not talking ok. I am driving to him right now, and you need to call the paramedics."

I hung up and my heart was racing fast, my hands shaking as I dialed Patrick's phone number.

"Sis, I don't feel OK!"

I hung up and called the paramedics right away.

"Hi, my name is Meriam and I just talked to my brother on the phone. He is alone in his apartment, and he has trouble talking. I think he's having a stroke. This is his address."

When I hung up, I told my colleagues what happened, closed my computer, and left the office. While I was rushing to the subway, I called Patrick again.

"Hawwooo"

"Patrick, please hang in there. The paramedics are on their way. Can you open the door?"

"I-can't-wwall"

I could hear the sirens of the ambulance while talking to Patrick, and I ran faster. It was a twenty-minute ride, but all I could think of was what I heard and that was anything but good. Yes, I was scared of what I just heard, scared of what I could expect. When I got out of the subway, I could hear the sirens of the fire trucks. I ran faster and when I arrived at Patrick's apartment on the fifth floor, the police were already there.

"Are you Meriam, the person who made the call?"

"Yes sir"

"Please, go inside, the paramedics are taking care of your brother."

My heart was racing like crazy, and Martin was also there. So were Patrick's adult twin girls and son. When I entered the apartment, I was not happy with what I saw. My brother was sitting on the floor and didn't look good at all. I lifted my thumb and he nodded as if he wanted to say: "thank you for being here for me." When the paramedics were done with Patrick, the fireman had to transfer him from the fifth floor into the ambulance. Because the stretcher didn't fit in the elevator of the building, they used a lift that was connected outside of the building to get Patrick downstairs and in the ambulance! Within one hour after Patrick called Martin, he was transferred to the ER of a nearby hospital. Later I understood that Patrick had called several family members to tell them that he wasn't feeling well.

Hours went by and around 8 PM, the neurologist came and told us that Patrick had a severe cerebral hemorrhage and was paralyzed on the right side of his body. Everybody was quiet. What did that mean? How severe was it? The only thing the neurologist could tell us is that the first 48 hours were critical. Patrick wasn't talking; we couldn't communicate with him. Everybody was sad and crying, but I was already organizing things in my mind. What if… nobody wanted to say the words, but what if Patrick could not talk or walk for the rest of his life? Can he stay in his apartment? He's single, so who will take care of him? What if he died?

I didn't sleep much that night. The next morning, I called the hospital to see how Patrick was doing and the nurse told me that he was very restless. He had fluid behind the lungs, was slurring his words and they were concerned about his health. It was less than twenty-four hours since the stroke and Patrick had high care nursing. Our family in Surinam knew of what had happened and our oldest sister had already sent some citrus fruits and fresh coconut oil with a close friend who was traveling from Surinam to the Netherlands.

Patrick has a lot of friends and the news spread very fast and some of them were visiting him. We could understand why, but we had to think of Patrick's health too. He couldn't talk, and he became very restless when they were in his room. I guess he didn't want them to see him in this situation and not being able to talk frustrated him. Patrick needed to rest to recover. We asked his friends to not visit him for a while and kept one friend up to date about his situation so that he could share the news with the rest of the friends. Forty-eight hours later Patrick's situation didn't improve. His arms and legs were swollen, and we were concerned about the fluid behind his lungs. But the citrus fruit and coconut oil from Surinam had arrived.

Our nephew and foster son (son of my late sister) and Patrick's ex-wife (mother of his kids) did a great job. They began to massage Patrick with the citrus fruit and coconut oil every day. Of course, after discussing this with the neurologist and other doctors. When they started with the massages, his body began to drain the excess fluids, and the nurses had to replace the urinary drainage bag more often. During the massages he was kicking his paralyzed arm and leg; it seems that the oil of the shell of the citrus fruit is stimulating the nerves. Patrick had a massage every day. Consistency is key! He started recovering slowly, but sometimes he didn't like the massage and would mumble something in Surinamese.

On November 18, 2012, it was Patrick's birthday. We celebrated it with him in the hospital; he slept most of the time but when we all stood in a circle and prayed, you could see the tears rolling down his cheek. That's when I knew he would be ok. He could hear us, but he couldn't say anything.

Two weeks went by, and the doctors told us that Patrick was talking gibberish. When I asked them what he was saying I realized he was talking Surinamese, and the Dutch doctors didn't know that. They were relieved and asked us to communicate with Patrick. He still didn't know our names, but he knew how we were related. The doctors found out that in contrast to what they previously thought, it was obvious that he was making improvements.

While Patrick was making progress, I felt the exhaustion, fear, anxiety coming up again. It reminded me of the time when I was running the whole day when Martin was on dialysis and in the hospital after surgery.

I took care of my brother, thankfully not alone, but I was also the caregiver of Martin. And I needed to take care of myself too.

I had promised myself that I would never burn out again! The mirror reminded me of my promise: "Meriam, what are you going to do for you?". And Martin reminded me too of what I had promised myself. Gotta love this guy!

While Patrick was out of the danger zone but still recovering in the hospital, I went on a 10-day Christmas cruise with Martin. To revitalize my energy, to do self-care, to love myself, and to spend time with my husband. I felt guilt coming up for a moment, but I waived it away as quickly as it came to my mind. Patrick was not alone, other family members also took care of him. Self-care is not selfish, it is needed!

Unfortunately, I was ill on Christmas Eve, but it only lasted for two days. I charged my battery and came back rejuvenated, and the result was that I could help Patrick even better.

After three weeks in the hospital, Patrick was transferred to a revalidation nursing home because he was still paralyzed. My nephew and his ex-wife continued with the massages every day during visiting time. Patrick stayed in this nursing home for five or six weeks and then he was ready for another revalidation home. In this home, he learned to move from his wheelchair to his bed within one day! He was active and the support of the family helped him get through this tough time. He had speech therapy, physio and every three or four weeks there was a consultation with the rehab doctor to discuss his improvements.

I remember one of the consults with Patrick. He started talking a bit but was still searching for the right words now and then. He could operate his wheelchair with his left arm, was feeling better, and was excited about his improvement.

But then.. the doctor told him:

"Patrick, you are doing much better, but I don't think that you will be able to walk anymore. Usually, people who have had such a severe stroke and were paralyzed, walk within a couple of weeks and you are still not walking after two months. I am so sorry."

Patrick looked at her and I could see him searching for words. After a few seconds, he said very slowly: I WILL WALK AND TALK AGAIN!

And he did! He took his first steps days later and I think that the doctor's words encouraged him to prove her otherwise. He was so committed to walking again and to taking care of his body.

When he started walking again the occupational therapist recommended looking for a safe place with facilities for someone who is partially disabled. And on June 18, 2013, we helped Patrick move to his new place where he still lives. Although his right arm doesn't function 100%, he is enjoying his "second" life to the max.

I am so grateful that it all went well, but when I was taking care of Patrick, I didn't take time to focus on my desire: the launch of my webshop.

It was a time of stress, exhaustion, and fear. I think it wasn't the right time to start.

Or was I procrastinating? When is the right time to do something?

Dear Caregiver,
Have you ever started with something and stopped because of caregiving? Did you find a moment or give yourself permission to continue?

In July 2013, I started with the preparation of launching a plus-size webshop again and I even tried to build the website on my own. I didn't succeed and asked my cousin who is a web designer to help me with building a website for Lady Plus Fashion.

I started my plus-size clothing webshop without having a fashion background. I was so determined to show the world that every(body) is beautiful no matter their size and I had success! Since 2013, I have worked with some interesting people e.g. the owner of the plus-size bridal shop in the Netherlands, an American television presenter and fashion designer who is mainly known for his work on wedding dresses, and a 4-time award-winning fashion designer. I also worked with a well-known designer from the USA who dressed a couple of famous plus-size actresses.

I went on national TV and I loved that the models were overloaded with compliments. I dressed several well-known women, and I was interviewed by a businesswoman. In that interview, I told my story: how I went from the girl who lived in a cozy home where her mom needed chewing gum to prevent her from getting wet when it rained to a businesswoman.

One of my other big wins was showing the world that every(body) is beautiful at the International Lymphoedema Framework Conference 2018 in the Netherlands.

> *Dear Caregiver,*
> *What is your biggest win in your life? I am proud of you!*

Remember I told you in the chapter Asking for Help about the question I received from the social worker in the hospital? There's a reason why I'm asking. Caregivers sometimes don't show their emotions to their care recipient.

Allow me to refresh your memory.

When Martin had his first kidney-pancreas transplant surgery I was still running from home to work, back home, took the car, went to the hospital, came back home late, and slept for a few hours a night. This went on for months without doing self-care. I was exhausted but I kept going.

I was a super-shero on an automatic pilot and I held up big for a long time. Martin was more than ready for Chapter 2.0, but his wife-to-be was not doing well.

We had a conversation with a social worker in the hospital. She first asked Martin how he felt both mentally and physically. Thankfully he felt better. Then she turned to me.

"Meriam, how are you doing?"

I was overwhelmed and before I knew it, I started crying and sobbing like a child. I cried for at least fifteen minutes and couldn't talk.

"Let it out Meriam. For whom have you been holding up big Meriam?"

Now I was mad at myself for showing others my vulnerability. They could see that I was tired, that I couldn't do it alone; that I was not OK.

When I was done crying, I apologized for using a whole box of Kleenex. Martin held my hand and said:

"hon, I am happy you finally showed what you have been hiding for so long. Let's work on this together. What if you take care of me and I take care of you?"

There went another box of Kleenex. I cried, sobbed, and felt angry because they saw the vulnerable Meriam. This super-shero was emotionally and physically on the ground. She thought she could do caregiving alone, but she thought wrong!

As I'm writing this, I am reliving that moment again!
Caregiver, please don't be like me!

I burnt out! When I heard the news from my doctor about my burnout my head was overloaded with questions:

"Oh no, how will I take care of Martin if something happens to me?"

"How can I get better asap so I can take care of him?"

"Wait, does this mean I have to take care of myself, me, Meriam?"

BOOM! Hello! Wake up!

So, thank you so much social worker for asking me how I was doing.

Dear Caregiver, how are you doing?
Breathe. You might want to punch me through the page.
That's ok. Can you catch yourself before you are burnt out?

When I got home, I sat alone in the living room; thinking about the conversation that was more of a cry session. Martin and the social worker saw my vulnerability, but I felt relieved. Wow, Meriam is human too!

I wanted to do something about my situation. Correction: I NEEDED to do something! I was in the darkness, but I had to find the courage to see the light bulb at the end of the tunnel.

"Are you crazy Meriam? Woman, let me tell you this: you are worthy of a wonderful life too! It's time you start thinking about YOU!"

There was no reason for me to stay in that unpleasant place.

I took a deep breath and all I could think of were those words.

"Get out of the darkness. You don't belong here! Can't you see the light? You will get there but you have to take action!"

I went upstairs to the bathroom and looked in the mirror.

"Meriam, what are you going to do for you?" To be honest, I couldn't answer. I looked in the mirror again and said:

"Meriam, what are you going to do for you? What if something happens to you? Who's going to take care of Martin? Name me one good reason why you ignore the signs of your body. Just one!". I could NOT answer.

I was tired, exhausted, and went to bed. The next day Martin and I had a conversation, and the result was that I left for a one-week break to Surinam. In that week, I thought of many things and did some self-care. I didn't know where to start, but I knew I needed to do something!

When I came back, I was still coping with burnout, but Martin and I had to prepare for the second major surgery. I was feeling a bit better after a week of breathing and thought I could start working full-time again, but I couldn't and had to call in sick. I was working at the Municipal Health Service and was thankful for the empathy of the colleagues. Some of them were doctors and they understood what I was going through. That was a relief as well. After all, I didn't have to worry or feel guilty because I called in sick. I thought that my exhaustion would be over in two or three days, but I guessed wrong. After two months I started working two hours a day and then slowly built it up until I could work full-time   again.

I learned my lesson. I didn't listen to my body when it was whispering, so it had to scream. I didn't listen to my gut when it told me that it would go wrong if I kept running from task to task.

I didn't tell my husband how tired I was. Why? Because he needed me, and I thought that I was a super-shero. I skipped that part of communication without realizing what effect it would have on us. I went over the edge and the result was burnout.

There's no one to blame except me. I ignored the signs of my body and if I wanted to change my life, I had to change my mindset. I had to use some techniques and tools. Asking for help, allowing myself to see possibilities, schedule and organize, do self-care, and love Meriam. Wow, I had to learn so much. That voice in my head kept talking to me.

"You got this! You can't quit now that you know that there's light at the end of the tunnel; you've come so far. I've got your back. You can do this!"

I started using the above techniques and tools slowly. I took baby steps. Overcoming the fear of asking for help and not playing small anymore. It wasn't easy, but if I wanted to transform my life, I had to. What did I have to lose? Nothing!

Dear Caregiver,
A friend of mine told me: please listen to your body when it's whispering, so it doesn't have to scream! Are you willing to listen to your body?

Sometimes we think that our me-time has been taken away. This only happens when you allow it to happen. I felt like this too. I didn't take time to breathe…

until I burnt out! In my head, I thought my me-time was taken away, but it wasn't. When I started scheduling and organizing, I created more time for myself.

Not having me-time affected my social life because I was always tired and too busy in my head. I started writing all doctor appointments in my calendar first and then I added the daily tasks. If I needed one hour to do something I would schedule an hour and fifteen minutes. Those fifteen minutes were breathing time for me. I started with scheduling per week.

Who takes care of the caregiver?

Caregivers are sometimes filled with guilt. But we also know that it wasn't anyone's fault. To be vigilant and wanting to be around someone 24/7 is a huge task. There is not much awareness about the struggles and needs of caregivers. Like any other individual, the caregiver needs to take care of himself/herself too. It's a tough job, it wasn't easy for me either but in the end, you have to take care of yourself. Give yourself permission to breathe and own your well-being. If YOU don't do it, nobody can or will do it for you. People might tell you to do self-care, but I recommend claiming your me-time and taking care of yourself as an individual and as a caregiver. Please don't say "I Can't" before you have given it a try, or before you have asked for help or scheduled to create time for yourself.

There is light at the end of the tunnel. Believe it!

When I do self-care, I feel that I show up for myself, that I am committed to myself. I also feel relaxed because I do something I love and enjoy. My self-care can vary from reading a book to listening to music or just doing nothing. Self-care is different for everybody, and it doesn't have to be a whole day in a spa. As much as I would love to, I can't be in the spa every day or every week or month. As long as you do something YOU love; it's self-care.

How do I take care of myself?

Once every 4 weeks, I go to the hairdresser. Every Saturday or Sunday I do a facial mask, hair mask, get my nails done, and I do a pedicure once a month; this is all done by myself. Martin and I have a typical Javanese massage every six weeks. This deep tissue massage helps me remove the toxin from my body and relaxes me too. My masseuse knows how to tackle the knots in my muscles; it hurts in the beginning but after a while, I feel relaxed; I can "breathe" again.

I love listening to music and that varies from breakfast jazz to Surinamese music. It depends on my mood.

Just sitting in the garden is also me-time for me. It's quiet where we live, especially during the daytime. I enjoy the birds (we have a bird's house attached to the shed), the dragonflies, the vegetables that grow, and flowers. When it is silent, things come to mind.

I also enjoy meditating for ten to fifteen minutes in the morning and evening. This is the time I claim for myself. Journaling is also one of my morning habits. While I enjoy my breakfast, I write whatever comes to mind for three to five minutes in my notebook. During the day, I do a quick breathing exercise by closing my eyes and taking five deep breaths. Visualizing what I would like to happen that day or in my life; ask my ancestors to give me the strength to reach my goals and tell myself that everything will be ok as long as I take action.

Dear Caregiver,
Can you name two things you love doing?

I find it hard to do self-care when I am busy and rescheduling my self-care moment comes to my mind. Please, don't do this! It's a big No! Self-care is needed and the negative chatter will always say:

"Meriam, you can reschedule and do self-care later."

Later means procrastinating! Please, don't do this! Caregivers often tend to put themselves last. I did it too because I was overthinking what others might think of me if I took time for myself. These thoughts made me feel guilty when I did self-care. Do not be like me!

Self-care is a practice and a commitment. After my burnout, I started doing self-care. Something bad had to happen first before I woke up! I supported myself by taking at least fifteen minutes per day to breathe. When I started doing that, I felt like I wanted more. Those fifteen minutes became twenty minutes, and twenty minutes became thirty minutes. At a certain point, I committed to taking 1 hour of me-time per day. That was my hour where I did something that made me relax and feel at ease. All of this didn't happen overnight. I had to take baby steps. But baby steps are steps too, right?

Dear Caregiver:
How do you support yourself?
You see, it's necessary to do self-care. You take care of your loved one but how do you take care of yourself?

Taking care of yourself is necessary and not selfish. Does the care recipient feel selfish about you taking care of him/her? Has the care recipient told you in his/her own words that you are selfish? I want to gently remind you that even hospitals don't give 24/7 care.

We are often overthinking. You don't have to ask for permission to take care of yourself! Look in the mirror and ask that beautiful person you see what will happen if he/she gets sick and can't take care of a loved one anymore. How would you feel? I think you already know the answer to this question but here it goes: "could you or do YOU want to prevent yourself from getting stress, exhaustion, burnout?" Be honest!

I know, it's not easy. This is a process, and it took me quite some time to learn. But I did it, and I feel so much better now that I don't feel selfish when taking care of myself. Not only that, but because I also take care of myself, I can be a better caregiver.

Boundaries

I love myself, and I do self-care regularly. I even schedule my self-care moments. It sometimes happens that Martin or Patrick asks me to help them with something. This can vary from helping them with cutting fingernails to calling insurance. If I have scheduled that time for myself, I tell them that I can help them, but at a later moment. If it's not urgent and life-threatening, my self-care moment is a priority. I expect them to do the same if I or somebody else asks them for help. If they have scheduled that time to do something they love, they should tell the other person that they can help, but at another time. It is ok to say no. Saying no to someone else is often saying yes to yourself.

Dear Caregiver,
Do you prioritize your self-care moment when there is no
urgency to help your loved one? Do you dare to say no?

Congratulations! You have started to strengthen the second S of your Personal Assistant SOS with an extra S (PASOSS).

Keep FOLLOW in mind.

Forgive yourself

Be **O**pen-minded

Listen to your gut

Learn new things

See and grab **O**pportunities

Know your **W**orth

SOCIAL CONNECTION

The 80+ couple that fills my cup

At first, I was resistant to cruising because of the idea that if something happened while being on the ocean, I couldn't get off the ship. Martin asked me several times to try it, and in February 2005 I gave it a shot and since then we have been cruising many times. At least once or twice a year. It is so relaxing, and the ocean breeze calms me. What I love about cruising is that you visit many places in a short time. It was the end of April 2015, when Martin and I took an amazing Caribbean cruise from Miami.

I remember that one evening at the beginning of the cruise, I went to the bar in the Atrium to order some drinks. It's such a beautiful spot and I always enjoy watching people who are dressed up or wearing casual styles having a great time. I stood at the bar and was almost ready to place my order when an elderly woman who was sitting on a chair beside me started coughing. She had choked on her drink.

"Are you ok? Can I get you a glass of water?"

"No honey, my martini will be just fine and help me," she said while coughing. And then she took a sip of her martini.

"See? It works just fine" with her voice still sore from coughing.

I looked at her and both of us laughed and we introduced ourselves. A couple of minutes later Martin and her husband joined us and the four of us started talking. There was a click, there was a connection.

Both of them are 80+ and enjoying life to the max. She's a beautiful woman, who takes care of herself and wears nice modern clothes. He is a handsome man, with a very pleasant voice and a great sense of humor.

"Where are you going for dinner," I asked them.

"We haven't decided yet." she said.

"Why don't you join us? We're going to the steak restaurant."

I can tell you that we had a wonderful time with this couple. We all felt so comfortable and talked about our families, health issues, and happy moments in our lives.

During the cruise, we had dinner together several times. One of the days was their wedding anniversary and I asked the restaurant manager to do something special for dessert and she got a rose from paperwork and there was a special anniversary cake made for them. It was so heartwarming to see them enjoy the attention, the care.

He had some health issues during the cruise, but thankfully everything went well. We spent as much time together as we could. This was the beginning of a long-term and long-distance relationship.

After the cruise, we stayed in touch via email and telephone. We have visited them several times since 2015, and we talk at least once or twice a week. In 2018, Martin and I visited them together with Patrick, my oldest sister from Surinam, and Martin's mom and sister. It was such a great time, and it felt like a family reunion even though they had met our family for the first time. On the last day of our holiday, Martin and I had planned a get-together. They brought pizza, and we enjoyed every single minute.

It was hard to say goodbye at the end of the evening. Do you know the feeling when you have to leave your loved ones who live thousands of miles away from you? It's a terrible feeling.

"When we left your place, we didn't talk for five minutes because of the lump in our throats" he wrote to me in his email the next day.

I will never forget these words. They fill my cup and I fill theirs. We are thousands of miles apart from each other, but we try to be there for them whenever they need us. In the years that we've known them, he had some surgeries. One of them was a nine-hour surgery. Thankfully she was not alone because their children and grandchildren take good care of them.

What I love about her is that even though she is 80+, she does self-care. She goes to the manicure, to the hairdresser and I do believe that it makes her feel pretty and gives her the strength, the power, both mentally and physically to take care of him. She asks for help when needed and she communicates with him.

I see many similarities between us that I admire: her determination, perseverance, and motivation. And I also see many character traits of him in Martin: funny, handsome but the most significant one is not giving up despite the illness! We talk about many things: from business ideas to health issues. I hang on their lips when they tell stories about their youth or when they were in their 20's and 30's.

"There is a reason why we met you. We meet so many people, but you and Martin are special to us. Thank you for being in our lives."

She often says this to us when we call and it's the truth; we meet a lot of people but not everybody stays in our life, and that's ok.

This 80+ couple has a special place in our hearts. We care, they care; there's an indescribable feeling of mutual love.

She is the caregiver for her husband, and he is her caregiver. As they get older both of them are struggling with health issues. When talking to them my first question is: "how are you both doing? How are you both feeling?"

I remember calling them one day in August 2020 and she picked up.

"He's in the hospital," she said. The ambulance took him at 2 A.M. and he wasn't feeling well Meriam." There was a vibration in her voice that worried me.

"Please, tell me what happened. I tried to call him via FaceTime, and he didn't answer. Now I know why" I said.

She told me that he reacted to one of those medicines he was taking. Of course, she was worried, and I listened to her. By listening to her, she could get it out of her head, off of her chest. I know that when I could tell my story and someone was just listening to me, it gave me relief.

Dear Caregiver,

If you take care of your elderly loved ones, have you ever asked them how they feel about you taking care of them? Honest communication is necessary. With this I mean, say what you feel, both mentally and physically. If you're tired, tell them; if you are happy, tell them.

If you find it hard to talk about something or feel sad, tell them. How do they fill your cup?

Fortunately, he went home a couple of days later and did much better. They both have health issues, and he does everything to help when she needs care. He would do the laundry or cooking so she can take care of herself to feel better. She is a role model for me; I imagine Martin and I in our 80's and taking care of each other as much as we can. I am so grateful for having these wonderful people in my life.

Doing self-care is important, and I enjoy seeing this 80+ lady treating herself to a manicure and making herself more beautiful. Having health issues doesn't have to mean that you can't be beautiful.

That's why, when one of my customers asked me in 2017 if I could help let the world see that plus-size women with Lymphoedema and Lipedema are beautiful too, I said "Yes" immediately. She was a board member of the Dutch Network for Lymphoedema and Lipedema. In summer 2018 the International Lymphoedema Framework (ILF) Conference would be held in the Netherlands. It would last for three days and the last day was planned for patients to meet suppliers who showed their new products.

On this day patients could also visit speaker presentations and workshops. The conference location was the former steamship SS Rotterdam; the first steamship of the Holland-America line between Rotterdam and New York. The ship was built in Rotterdam. The legendary former flagship of the Holland

America Line is rich in history and renowned for its cultural and historic value. In one word: Beautiful!

My customer told me that she would like to organize a fashion show for Patients Day and asked me if I was willing to show the world that plus-size women with lymphoedema and lipedema can be bold and beautiful too.

I was thrilled with the idea. It was almost a year away from the day she asked me, but I could imagine those beautiful women walking on the catwalk in their compression garments and our outfits. I wanted to take care of these beautiful women.

A few weeks before the date my cousin, who was a stylist, and I planned a meet and greet session at my home. We also wanted the women to try some outfits and were in luck because there was also a makeup artist who was a close friend of my customer. There were four models in the US sizes 12 – 22/24.

It was a blast. Imagine eight women in a living room, trying different styles and having fun. I loved to see what the outfits, mostly dresses, did to the models. They felt beautiful and most important: confident. They were ready to show the world that even though they had to wear compression sleeves and socks they were BEAU-TI-FUL. Their appearance was amazing. We tried several styles until we could make a final decision on who should wear what outfit on that day. From casual to date-night to evening style. We would end the show with an amazing wedding gown from my friend who owned a plus-size bridal shop.

On Patients Day, we arrived early in the morning. The fashion show started at noon and the models were super excited. They couldn't wait to show the attending patients that they are beautiful too.

The makeup artist started as soon as she could, and my cousin and I started sorting out the outfits per model. The fashion show was for all sizes including men, but we were dressing only the plus-size women. When it was time to go on the catwalk, there was some nervousness in the models. They had to take the stairs to go down to the catwalk, which went all the way to the hall where the suppliers had their stands. Some of the suppliers were the sponsors of the compression garment.

I remember that the models with other sizes went first. The crowd, almost three hundred patients, were excited and we could hear the cheering from our room upstairs. When our first model came on the catwalk, I was still in the room getting the other models ready. I remember hearing someone yell: "OMG, look how beautiful she is".

The crowd went crazy and started clapping and cheering on the model. Someone told me later that the model's mom who was in the crowd was crying when she saw how people reacted to her daughter. The second model hit the catwalk and I could hear the encouragement. Then the third and the fourth model hit the catwalk. Oh my… I went to take a quick look and I got goosebumps. The room was filled with love, tears, encouragement, confidence. Yes! Together with my cousin, I took care of these beautiful women. We were able to let them show their inner and outer beauty and boost their confidence!

The models were dressed in stylish jeans, shirt, and kinky flower jacket and compression socks; a black lace dress with one compression glove and pink compression socks (Yes! very cool), a beautiful black and white faux wrap dress with black compression socks and red shoes (the crowd loved this bold combination!) and a plum wrap dress with a sweetheart neckline with skin color compression socks and arm socks!

"Yass, we are beautiful too", "OMG woman, you look amazing", "Wow, I've never seen you in a dress", "You should wear dresses more often", "Oh wow, that jacket and jeans look very stylish on you".

My cousin had tears in her eyes.

"We nailed it, auntie."

"Yes we did, and this is only the casual style. I wonder how the crowd will react if they see the next round."

The second and third rounds were amazing. The models were more excited and confident after the first round to show the crowd how wonderful they looked in the A-line teal and bronze-gold/black lace dresses, the wrap dresses with feminine floral prints, and abstract blue/white prints. All dresses were paired with their compression garment.

Yes, having Lymphoedema or Lipedema doesn't mean that you are ugly or unattractive!

The crowd went wild and wanted more of our models, but we only had half an hour to show some styles. Then it was time for the showstopper: the wedding gown! At first, we decided that my customer, the board member, would be the showstopper. But on the first day of the conference, she received a phone call from home. She had to leave the conference to take care of her three-year-old daughter who is a diabetic and had health problems. This mommy is a badass caregiver and took good care of her little girl.

One of the other models was willing to be the showstopper, but she had another size, and we had no time to fit a wedding dress before the show. We took her measurements and I sent them to my friend, the owner of the bridal shop. Her daughter brought one wedding dress and guess what: it was perfect!

This 5'8 ft model had a no-nonsense attitude with her dark brown hair, and US size 16. When she came down the stairs in the wedding gown, you can already guess what happened. I thought I was at the Oscars when I saw all the flashing of the cameras. She wore a beautiful strapless wedding gown with a veil. Yes, plus-size women with Lymphoedema and Lipedema are beautiful too!

Our mission was accomplished: together with my cousin, the makeup artist, the board member, and the models I showed the world that Every(body) is Beautiful.

The models received so many compliments, and this boosted their self-confidence. I am so grateful and honored that I had the opportunity to take care of them in a different way. The results are still visible to the present date. When you feel beautiful you may feel happy, strong, bold! And that's exactly what I saw on that day. Not only with the models, but also the crowd. They saw that there were possibilities to be beautiful, even with their lymphoedema and/or lipedema. At that time, I didn't realize what type of caregiving I was providing. I am so grateful that I could contribute to this event, to this feeling of being beautiful and happy, to get those women out of their comfort zone. There's no need to feel unattractive or ugly when you -according to society- look "different" than others!

Testimonials of two models:

When I met Meriam, I was very excited about the opportunity to work with her. Our paths crossed in a period of my life where I was very conscious of my physical appearance. I was used to hiding my insecurities underneath my bubbly and outgoing personality. I had just finished a personal development training and she helped me to translate my newly learned skills into a professional yet approachable appearance. I cherish the warm memories and still hear her advice playing in the back of my mind once in a while.

Thank you, Meriam, for showing me my hidden inner beauty!

Because of my lipedema, I was very self-conscious about my body, especially about my legs. Wearing a dress has been out of the question since my teens. And that did harm my self-esteem and the way I viewed myself. And then I met Meriam. The way she looks at life, the way she carries herself, how she dresses.... it was catchy. She is such a kind and loving person. She showed me that shifting my focus from my 'worst' to my best and most of all how she can make me see the best of me..... it made me feel confident, feminine! To be able to sparkle from the inside out.... she helped me make that possible again!

Meriam rocks!

Thank you, ladies, for filling my cup. You gave me the knowledge and strength to serve customers with problems in the areas of lymphoedema and lipedema. You gave me and others the confirmation AGAIN that every(body) is beautiful and the opportunity to care for you differently. Thank you!

Dear Caregiver,
Do you ever buy yourself some nice clothes and put on some makeup? If so, how do you feel? Does feeling beautiful fill your cup as well?

When I connect socially, I forget caregiving for a moment. I focus on the stories of friends or family and it's nice to be "busy" with something other than caregiving.

Social connection means learning from others, no matter the subject. And breathing while you are with others.

I sometimes find it hard to make social connections when I think of the idea that Martin will be alone at home. Although he is totally fine now, there will always be a thought in my mind: "will he be fine". I wouldn't call it fear, more concern. And when I ask him if he'll be fine, he confirms. This makes it so much easier for me. Martin enjoys being alone. It's his me-time and he usually listens to music or reads a book. He does self-care.

The time I didn't have a social connection but should have was when Martin was recovering in the hospital. I was running from one task to another and didn't allow myself to have a social life. There were plenty of people in my community who invited me for lunch or dinner, but I didn't accept the invitations because I insisted on being with Martin in the hospital every day. Spending more time with him was a feeling that I was in control. But I wasn't. I was losing control because it wore me out, so instead of giving me energy, it was eating up my energy.

Social connection is a practice and a commitment. In the beginning, I felt guilty. One day I finally went for dinner with a friend while Martin was recovering in the hospital. He had four or five visitors, so he was with more people than I was, and I still felt guilty. I was looking at my phone constantly. My friend knew about my situation and understood what I was going through. After going for a drink or visiting friends for the 3rd or 4th time, that guilt started fading away and I could finally enjoy the moment.

Dear Caregiver,
Do you have a social life? If not, why not?
"I can't" is not allowed as an answer.

There was a time in my life when I believed I could not have a social life. And this was all a lie! There were days when I was caught up in lies that I didn't know were lies. I can't get that time back, but I wish I had been open to the truth earlier. It is hard to see the lies in the middle of sorrow.

Congratulations! You have started to strengthen the last S of your Personal Assistant SOS with an extra S (PASOSS).

Keep FOLLOW in mind.

Forgive yourself

Be **O**pen-minded

Listen to your gut

Learn new things
See and grab **O**pportunities
Know your **W**orth

REVIEW AND REIMAGINE

If you feel like you are struggling, ask yourself these questions:

1. Do you love yourself? If so, name two ways of how you show it within fifteen seconds.
2. Who will take care of your loved one if something happens to you?
3. Name one good reason why you are ignoring the signs of your body.

When I feel like I'm getting too tired, I look in the mirror and ask myself these three questions. And I say my favorite affirmation:

I Am Worthy Of A Wonderful Life Too!

The questions and affirmation are my barometer and help me prevent burnout. They helped me see my personal growth.

I have been a caregiver now for more than twenty years. And I have learned the hard way that:

- self-love doesn't make me an egoist
- self-care is a must

- communication is necessary and required to avoid misunderstandings and to have clarity for both me and my loved one

- scheduling and organizing creates time for me to breathe

- asking others for help is not a shame or a sign of weakness

- I was not alone; even though it felt that way sometimes

The difference between taking care of Martin and Patrick is that when I was taking care of Martin, I didn't use the techniques and tools that could save me from burning out. When I took care of Patrick, I was more structured, more aware of self-care, more organized and the result was that I could both enjoy my life, stay in my power while taking care of him. With Patrick, I listened to my body when it was whispering. I didn't let it scream.

My gifts with caregiving have wonderfully transformed me over time. I noticed that I love myself more every day. I do more self-care, even if it's for only ten minutes and I can say "No" without feeling guilty. I schedule my self-care moments and when someone asks me to do something for them, I can say no and offer help at another time. Saying "No" to someone else is saying "Yes" to Meriam.

I do respect the question and I will always offer an alternative. If Patrick asks me to take him somewhere on a specific day and I have already scheduled that day to practice self-care I would say:

"I can't on that day or time, but I can bring you on this day or that time." I also noticed that I was helping other caregivers when I saw that they were falling into the same trap I did when caring for Martin. I empowered them to do what I did years ago to be able to stay in their power and harmony.

It is such a relief when you take care of someone and know that you have time to breathe, time for yourself.

I am worthy of a wonderful life too, and it's ok to have moments for myself to breathe. Please permit yourself to own your well-being. Say "No" when it's needed, and don't feel guilty when you can't do what others ask of you.

Caregivers who love themselves, permit themselves to see possibilities, ask for help, schedule, organize, do self-care, socialize and communicate well with the one they take care of, will be able to own their well-being. I appreciate them so much for what they are doing!

Keep FOLLOW in mind.

Forgive yourself

Be **O**pen-minded

Listen to your gut

Learn new things

See and grab Opportunities

Know your Worth

CONCLUSION:

Caregiving is a service and a mission.

I take baby steps; I walk before I run. Some of those steps include journaling for three to five minutes in the morning and meditating for only ten minutes. Sometimes, those steps require me to move forward, and sometimes those steps require me to look in the mirror and say: "I am worthy of a wonderful life too!"

The way I maintain momentum is that I give myself compliments for what I have accomplished. I have come through a lot, and I am proud of myself for not quitting on Martin, Patrick, and myself and the love between us.

Martin always tells me that I was his vine he was hanging on. In those tough times, he was so busy taking care of himself and noticed too late that his wife was burning out. He is so grateful that I was his caregiver and thanks me for that. He recovered from many surgeries, and I recovered from the burnout. Both of us were forced to do self-care together and apart, communicate better, and set boundaries.

Most of what happened with Martin helped me when Patrick needed caregiving. He always says that he is grateful that I called the paramedics right away. He is also grateful for the help and the love he still gets from me and the family. He realized that it wasn't easy for any of us. Sometimes he didn't want to ask for help because he didn't want to be a burden, but I told him that he should not think for me or others. If I can't help him when he wants it, we can always look for other possibilities. Just like Martin and I, Patrick was also forced to do self-care, communicate better, and set boundaries.

Own your well-being.

Dear Martin,

We have been together now for almost twenty-three years. In those years we have been through many happy moments but also sad and scary moments. We have traveled a lot, met many inspiring people from all over the world and we continue to do so.

You are one in a million. What I admire most about you is how you have coped with your illness. You've been a diabetic since you were fifteen years old, suffered from kidney failure, been on dialysis, and finally, you had a kidney-pancreas transplant. You've had so many surgeries that I lost count. It takes a lot of strength, both mentally and physically to carry such a burden. But you did it!

You taught me how to love someone unconditionally and how to take care of someone you love without losing hope. Because of you, I was taught that doing self-care is not selfish but needed, that asking for help is ok, and that I can't do caregiving alone. I didn't listen to my body and unfortunately, you had to see me burn out while caring for you. But you didn't let me stay in that dark place. We leaned on each other and got out of there together.

I admire your generosity; we don't have kids of our own, but you agreed to offer my nephew and cousin from Surinam a safe home to get their higher education diplomas and find out who they are as a person. I also learned from you why I should travel: meeting, connecting, respecting, and understanding people with different cultures from all over the world contributed to my personal development.

Your right mindset regarding your illness got you through the most difficult time of your life, and I am so grateful that I was and still am a part of that lesson. I learned how it feels to be helpless and powerless. But the most important thing I learned is that there is a way to make a change.

At the time I hated the tough lessons, but now I realize that they have transformed me into the person who I am today: Caregiver 2.0!

I want to thank you from the bottom of my heart because it's not only me that will benefit from what I've learned from you.

Love you so much.

-Your wife Meriam

First of all, a shout out to family caregivers!

I am grateful that I got a second chance from God. I've been in a dark place. I had a stroke, couldn't remember the names of my kids and family, and couldn't walk or talk. I was captured in my own body!

At first, I wanted to give up. I prayed to God every day to take me. I couldn't do anything myself and I didn't want to ask for help because I didn't want to bother anyone.

Living like this was no option for me; I just wanted to die. When the doctor told me that I would not be able to walk anymore I was devastated. But my family never gave up on me and their support and belief in me gave me the power to move forward. I told the doctor that -no matter what- I would walk and talk again. And I did!

I do realize that I will never be the same again, but I can live on my own and do a lot myself again.

My gratitude to everyone who supported me is beyond words.

Thank you from the bottom of my heart.

I love you; I appreciate you,
Patrick

P.S.

Who do you belong to?

I belong to the Universe. Why? Because I Ask, I Believe, and I Receive. That's what the Universe does, and I am so grateful that now I see how it works. I'm not there yet, I don't know everything but what I do know is that I can and will help others in a way I can.

I Ask, I Believe, I Receive.

About the Author

Meriam Boldewijn is a devoted wife, inspiring author, caregiver advocate, motivational speaker, and business entrepreneur. She is the founder and proud owner of both Caregiver 2.0, a 6-week online program that offers support, coaching, and life skills to caregivers all over the world, and Lady Plus Fashion, a former webshop in exclusive plus-size women's clothing (2013-2019).

If you enjoyed this book and need more guidance in the area of owning your well-being as a caregiver, I'm inviting you to join my coaching program Caregiver 2.0. You can find more info via

www.meriamboldewijn.com

As a result of this coaching program, caregivers who spend their lifetimes helping family members or patients learn how to prevent or overcome burnout from taking care of everyone else. They reduce stress, release the guilt and shame of sometimes putting themselves first, and they now implement a simple strategy when the thought comes to their mind: Why me! Caregivers can prioritize themselves as number one first which can extend their quality of life, so they can breathe better, live more and finally help everyone in their circle from a place of their overflow.

Connect with us:

Instagram: Meriam Boldewijn

Facebook: Hellomeriam

Twitter: Meriam Boldewijn

Clubhouse: Meriam Boldewijn

YouTube: Meriam Boldewijn

RESOURCES

Ashley Jackson-Thompson: www.timelessdreamevents.com

Avis Adele Tullo hitchcock: www.facebook.com/radicalcarepodcast

Jessica Lizel Cannon: www.jessicalizelcannon.com

Julia Cameron: *The Artist's Way*

Lisa Nichols: www.motivatingthemasses.com

Marina Rieboldt-O'Neill: www.cognitivevitality.net

Dr. Sarah Jefferis: www.sarahjefferis.com

Made in United States
North Haven, CT
06 November 2021